THE MAGIC OF
MENTAL DIAGRAMS

THE MAGIC OF MENTAL DIAGRAMS

EXPAND YOUR MEMORY, ENHANCE YOUR CONCENTRATION,
AND LEARN TO APPLY LOGIC

CLAUDIO AROS

Psychologist and Life Coach

Translated by Gladis Castillo

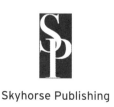

Skyhorse Publishing

Original title: **GUÍA PARA LA CREACIÓN DE DIAGRAMAS MENTALES**
© Claudio Aros, 2006

© Editorial Océano, SL (Barcelona, Spain)
Illustrations: Paula Leiva
Images: Oceano Ambar archive

English translation © 2015 by Skyhorse Publishing

Skyhorse Publishing books may be purchased in bulk at special discounts for sales promotion, corporate gifts, fund-raising, or educational purposes. Special editions can also be created to specifications. For details, contact the Special Sales Department, Skyhorse Publishing, 307 West 36th Street, 11th Floor, New York, NY 10018 or info@skyhorsepublishing.com.

Skyhorse® and Skyhorse Publishing® are registered trademarks of Skyhorse Publishing, Inc.®, a Delaware corporation.

Visit our website at www.skyhorsepublishing.com.

10 9 8 7 6 5 4 3 2 1

Library of Congress Cataloging-in-Publication Data is available on file.

Cover design by Qualcom Designs
Cover photo credit Thinkstock

ISBN: 978-1-63220-328-1
Ebook ISBN: 978-1-63220-861-3

Printed in China

Contents

Integrating what has been learned

Applications

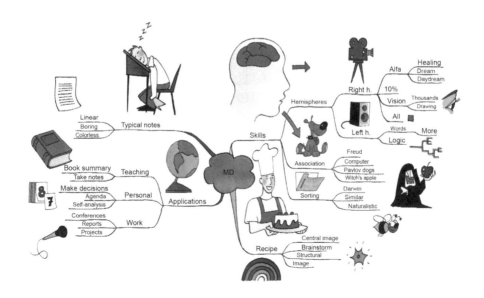

1 Introduction:
The wonderful world
of mental diagrams

- School days

- Preliminary findings based on my notes

- There is always light at the end of the tunnel

- Getting started

- A thorough analysis

- What you will be able to obtain from mental diagrams

■ School days

I remember that when I was a college student I overheard one mother tell another how her son was putting forth a lot of effort in studying and yet he was barely getting by in school. Obviously, the conversation got my attention because my case was very similar: I put in a lot of effort and got little result. The distraught mother painfully explained that every afternoon her son would return home after spending all day in school and then proceeded to spend five or six hours (or even nights, she said) studying. The woman said there were pages and pages of very neat notes. I thought it was strange that he had very neat notes, and I came to the conclusion that the poor guy spent his afternoons rewriting the notes he took in the morning. Spending hours and hours rewriting notes neatly is arduous and exhausting. Instead of spending valuable time studying, he was rewriting notes, which was no guarantee for good grades.

At that moment I did some soul-searching. At least that guy had neat notes, but I . . . you could say that I had something resembling notes. What exactly did I have? A series of incomplete papers written in unintelligible script (which I still have) with rivers of runaway words. In fact, to be honest, I never reviewed them because I did not think they were very reliable. To me they were silent enemies that did not want to make things easier for me. Our relationship was such that they did not understand me and I did not understand them. To understand this mystery, I will explain in a few words how I spent my time in the classroom on any given day: we sat down, the professor talked for an hour, we wrote everything he said, and an hour later the class ended with us murmuring and looking very tired. Multiply this by eight daily classes and by six years, and you will get a pretty good picture of what it took me to earn a university degree. Personally, after a day like that, I was left with a stiff hand, and the last thing that would ever cross my mind would be to spend my evenings rewriting my messy notes.

■ Preliminary findings based on my notes

In a quest to find a solution to my problem I decided to look into what was wrong with my despised notes. After an in-depth investigation, I came to four basic conclusions:

1st conclusion. There were no clear ideas

When jotting down directly what the teacher said, I did not grasp the main idea nor did I know where he was going with his lecture. Those ideas were present, but they were buried in an ocean of words. Trying to find the main ideas was archeological work and often the results were fruitless or I came to erroneous conclusions. The sea of words obscured the main idea.

2nd conclusion. Every page looked the same

I also discovered that if the pages were not numbered, it was very easy to confuse them with each other since they were very similar. Imagine facing a lot of garbled words and spotty pages all written with the same ink: it is scary. I remember I eagerly tried to defeat those notes and wrestle the main ideas, but I almost always lost out to their hypnotic effect. Yes, while reading all those pages that were so similar and had so little meaning I would go into a kind of trance, so that when I got to the third page I realized that I was still automatically reading without comprehending. In those moments, I stopped to make myself tea and start the second part of the battle, but when I returned, the pages continued to have that terrible hypnotic ability. In short, I can say that those pages were endowed with the power of monotony and boredom.

3rd conclusion. **I was wasting a lot of time sorting through the notes**

For starters, I had taken more notes than necessary so I had to do a first reading to see that the words made sense. In a second reading I tried to separate the wheat from the chaff, and finally I did one more reading to see if I had forgotten anything. The problem was not that I had to do three readings to study but that I had to do three readings just to see what was in those notes!

4th conclusion. **It was drudgery**

The task of sorting through notes in search of intelligent life was an arduous task. I often imagined the work of gold prospectors who had to stand for hours in an icy river sorting through pebbles in the hope of finding the gold nugget that would solve all their problems (well, actually, even if they found it immediately they went to the nearest town and spent it on all kinds of pleasures, so the following week they were back to kneeling in the cold river looking for more nuggets).

In my case, the gold nuggets would not take me to a world of pleasure; instead they were the beginning of my ordeal and the first step that brought me closer to seriously considering dropping out. I do not know if you ever experienced the frustrating feeling of doing a job that makes no sense and the feeling of wasting hours of your precious life.

Dramatic consequences

However, I did not stop there in examining the poor quality of my notes. I wanted to get to the consequences. Based on my own experience I knew that somehow it affected my motivation, and I found that my emotions and even my attention were affected. These are the consequences I discovered:

- Understandably, I lost my concentration because the information was incomprehensible (lack of attention)
- I lost my eagerness to learn (lack of motivation)
- The harder I tried, the less I progressed (and generated negative feelings)
- You can get into the habit of making notes of notes, so a lot of time and effort is wasted

■ There is always light at the end of the tunnel

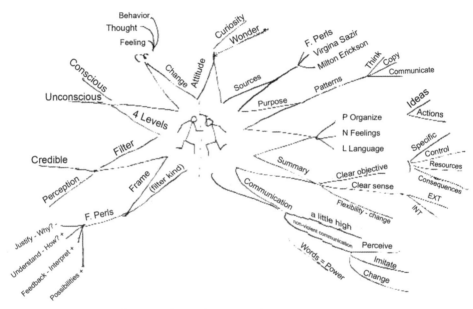

Sample mental diagram regarding neuro-linguistic programming

Back in those days, I studied a course on advertising. The professor explained that good advertising campaigns could be made through a simple combination of key words, illustrations, and colors. And looking at the different campaigns and reports that companies made, I wondered if notes could be written in a more appealing and clear manner. I explained to some of my classmates the idea of compiling our notes into a colorful document with pictures. As you can imagine, this idea was welcomed with laughter and one of my peers told me that if the professor were to see such a thing, I would fail the course. Well, I have always been aware that one does not succeed on the first attempt, but I believed that another format was needed to assimilate so much information; moreover, all the science of advertising (so to speak) backed up my idea from afar. And I do not remember very well, but somehow I got the chance to see a mental diagram, which was a revelation. It was incredible, a clear structure of a sociology topic with colors and drawings! I know I may seem flippant, but it was just what I had been looking for and they were called mind maps. Those two words completely hooked me and said it all, so without any hesitation I went to the nearest bookstore and asked for a book on mental diagrams. To my surprise there was more than one, and I chose one whose author had a curious name: Tony Buzan.

TONY BUZAN, THE PIONEER

When I was a sophomore in college, a young Tony Buzan decided to understand how the brain works to be able to maximize its use. He was disappointed when in the library he was told that there were no books on this topic. Given the perplexity of having hundreds of books about the brain's physiology and mechanism but not a single book that helped promote these concepts, he promised himself to correct this injustice. Thus, with more courage than knowledge, he entered into the stormy world of learning. According to him, he plunged into an unknown territory on which he built a powerful technique that has lasted over twenty years: mind maps.

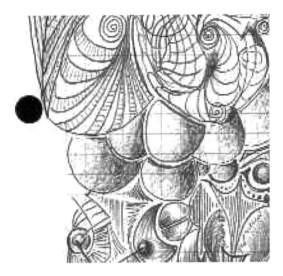

*Geometric figure made by a student in
literature class*

In life there are a number of things that are not taught in schools and which are essential to function. Usually teachers do not teach us an effective note-taking method. As a business school professor and professional trainer I cannot help but look at the notes taken by my students and assistants. I see that most of them repeat exactly the same mistakes that I made, or their notes are so dense or so telegraphic that they are incomprehensible. Also, they are so unattractive that it is almost impossible to look back at them or at least look at them fondly. Still, I often find drawings in them, but they are never usually related to the subject at hand (stars, squares, and all kinds of geometric shapes).

Could there be some note-taking method that could save us time, give us clarity, and be simple to practice? Is there something that could help us organize information easily while also look nice? Yes, such a method exists: it is the famous method of mental diagrams. And this book is designed to show it to you. You probably already guessed that the book was about mental diagrams (since it is on the cover of the book), but you cannot begin to fathom all the different areas where you can apply this revolutionary technique.

■ Getting started

Mental diagrams are not only designed to help students with their note-taking. Their uses are much wider and even reach the field of business. This technique has been applied very successfully in various companies. A good example is a chemical company that had a problem with competitiveness. This company manufactured a wide range of products applied to such diverse fields as the energy and telecommunications industries. The success of this company depended on marketing the most innovative products in the shortest time possible because the competition was always at its heels. Its quick innovation depended on clear and concise communication and on effective collaboration between different departments to solve problems quickly. How could they be more competitive and shorten the time to launch new products?

The head of research and development explained it this way: ". . . it is very difficult to start an R&D project if you are not very sure of the tasks that need to get done, who should do them, and who has to be involved in the project. Our starting point is always a state of confusion that is sometimes hard to get out of; to be more competitive we needed another way of working, but which one?" In this case, they were lucky that this leader accidentally attended a course about mental diagrams. The idea seemed interesting and he decided to apply the technique to their projects. As he explained, "Why not? I had nothing to lose and it might even help me . . ." The success of this new technique in their work is hard to explain, but in his words, ". . . before, in order to define a project, we had to have many long and frustrating meetings that got out of hand more than once. Now, in one single meeting we can have a clear and definite picture of the entire project. Isn't that amazing?" Also there were other advantages that were initially unnoticed, such as planning a structured agenda: ". . . one of the unexpected results was saving time in meetings. Currently many of them last only half an hour. Everyone takes a diagram of all the project ideas, actions, and related documents. The diagrams become agendas for future meetings."

The case of this chemical company is not unique in the business market. Some others that have already implemented the mental diagrams method say:

"The biggest benefit of mental diagrams is that we have participatory meetings in which we easily find the best ideas and quickly put them into action. It represents a new way of thinking and collaborating."
DFS Group Vice President

"Thanks to mental diagrams I can spend more time on the project and less time on administrative tasks such as transcribing meeting notes, defining the project's details, or creating reports that I send to my supervisor."
PMP Project Manager

"Through mental diagrams, we redesigned the entire retail department in just three meetings. When we looked at all the work we accomplished we realized how productive this really was."
IBC Marketing Manager

"Mental diagrams are a unique tool for someone like me who has to constantly assimilate and process information from various sources."
JG, M4 consulting partner

"Companies call us because we can understand problems and provide solutions. Mental diagrams help us approach the problem with the client because it is an easy way to address problems. Using mental diagrams we save a great amount of time, and time is money."
SKR Consulting

■ A thorough analysis

Several years ago I had a job-related question. A twenty-nine-year-old man wanted to know what kind of work suited him best, both with regard to his professional skills as well as his personality profile. He explained that he had spent the last eight years of his working life in car sales. Those eight years had brought him success and prestige, yet he felt he wanted to do something else, or at least he thought he was qualified to do other type of work. Under normal circumstances I would have followed the established protocol for such cases. I would have begun by administering a series of intelligence, aptitude, and personality tests. After analyzing them, I would have interviewed him thoroughly and at the end, I would have rendered some kind of report. However, this time I thought I should try a different course of action and I remembered the mental diagrams technique. Could it be applied to counsel a job seeker? The truth is that I had never before utilized it in a case like this, but it seemed appropriate due to its ease of use. More importantly, this young salesman needed good self-analysis as opposed to a bunch of tests.

Without too much hesitation, I suggested approaching the problem from a different angle and the young man gladly accepted. The mental diagrams about his life took us less than two hours to make. At the end, he proudly saw his life, skills, traits, needs, and motivations, all on one sheet. Colors, patterns, and even some tears were reflected coherently and orderly in the diagram. After looking at it for several minutes he seemed very satisfied and said, ". . . this is what I was really looking for."

Subsequently, I delved into applying mental diagrams to personal matters, and I was surprised by its many good uses. Accordingly, I added mental diagrams to my personal toolbox. But I will explain these applications to you further on.

■ What you will be able to obtain from mental diagrams

So far I have given you some examples of how mental diagrams can be applied. If you were paying attention, you noticed that we covered three major functional areas. The first was related to education, the second to the field of business, and the third to personal issues. However, I have provided just a few examples of their application. Their use goes beyond taking notes or managing projects. Mental diagrams are a way of **organizing large blocks of information coherently for our brain**. As such, you will find that mental diagrams create a unique, creative, and simple synthesis out of complex elements. And therein lies the power of mental diagrams.

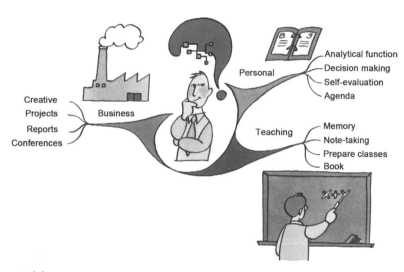

Applying mental diagrams

BENEFITS OF MENTAL DIAGRAMS

Mental diagrams can help you:

- be more creative.
- save time.
- concentrate.
- organize and clarify ideas.
- remember.
- plan.
- study more and better.
- see things as a whole.

And above all, they help you save trees because less paper is needed as compared to other methods.

WHAT ARE THE ONLY THINGS YOU NEED TO LEARN THIS TECHNIQUE?

- a blank sheet
- pencils and colored markers
- your brain
- your imagination
- this book, of course

Basic skills

To make mental diagrams you need to understand **how the brain works** (Ch. 2) and know its basic skills.

- The first is **control of the right hemisphere**. This hemisphere is related to visualization (Ch. 3) and space (Ch. 4).

- The second skill **is related to the left hemisphere** and words (Ch. 5).

- The third skill is related to **associations established in the brain** (Ch. 6).

- And the fourth refers to **how we structure the world** (Ch. 7).

Once these brain skills are understood and exercised, we can start **creating mental diagrams** in the second section.

2 Anatomy of our minds: Two brains are better than one

What would you say if I told you that we have two different minds and not just one? And if I were to add that all your school years focused on developing just one of these minds while the other was completely ignored?
Is it possible to use these two minds to their full potential?

In this chapter we will review the most revolutionary scientific theories about brain function, find clues about how mental diagrams work, and learn the functions of each of these powerful minds.

- **We only use 10 percent of our mind**

- **Case WJ 1961**

- **Anatomy of a human brain**

- **I hear a voice inside of me**

- **Two is better than one**

■ We only use 10 percent of our brain

The decade of the nineties was declared "Decade of the Brain" by the United States Congress. But why? It was due to great advances in research that in just a few years made it possible to realize things that were once considered science fiction. Even now we continue to be immersed in an exciting period of discoveries in psychology.

Albert Einstein, our beloved genius, somehow predicted our limited mental development: "We only use 10 percent of our mind's potential," he once remarked. But one needs to clarify that some authors claim that this percentage is too generous. In view of this statement one can only wonder what the hell the rest of the brain is doing. Would it be possible to use the remaining 90 percent for any practical purpose?
The answer could not be more straightforward: yes, with the appropriate techniques and knowledge we can increase the brain's potential.
But before driving the Formula 1 car that is your brain, you will have to learn a little about its mechanics. You will have to become familiar with certain concepts such as inner dialogue, consciousness, and hemispheres or states of mind. These ideas are not at all complicated, and you will be able see their practical application through mental diagrams.
If you are willing to look into the inner workings of the brain, keep reading about the interesting findings by the young student Gazzaniga.

■ Case WJ 1961

A particularly exciting part of the study of the brain began in 1961, when Roger Sperry became interested in a forty-eight-year-old veteran whose head was hit by shrapnel during World War II.

A few years after his injury, WJ (as we will call the war veteran) started having seizures; they became so frequent and so severe that no remedy could control them. He would fall unconscious and start foaming at the mouth, often injuring himself. Doctors tried different medications unsuccessfully for more than five years. At last, surgeons sectioned off part of his brain, the corpus callosum, and his epilepsy ceased as if by magic. There was a difficult recovery period, during which WJ, a man of above normal intelligence, could not speak, but after a month he announced that he felt much better than in recent years. He seemed unchanged in his personality and perfectly normal.

Meanwhile, Sperry had convinced a graduate student named Michael Gazzaniga to perform a series of tests on WJ. The young graduate student quickly discovered some very strange things in his patient. To begin, WJ could carry out verbal commands ("Raise your hand," "Bend your knee") only on the right side of his body. He could not respond with his left side. When WJ was blindfolded, he could not even tell which part of his body was touched if it happened on his left side.
In fact, as the testing continued, it became increasingly difficult to think of WJ as a single person. Unaware, his left hand did things that the right hand

refused. He once threatened his wife with the left hand, while the right hand was trying to help her and bring the belligerent hand under control.

Gazzaniga remembers that he was playing horseshoes with WJ in the patients' courtyard when suddenly WJ lifted an ax with his left hand. Alarmed, Gazzaniga quickly left the scene: "The right hemisphere might have gotten angry and had taken control of the ax . . . I did not want to become a victim of this experiment so I decided to leave." Through other tests, he discovered that only the left half could speak. The right remained silent forever, unable to perform tasks requiring judgment or language-based interpretation. Indeed, the first tests that WJ underwent seemed to show that his right hemisphere was practically nonexistent. But the day came when WJ, with a pencil in his left hand, was shown the outline of a Greek cross. Swiftly and without hesitation, he copied it, drawing the whole figure with one continuous line. But when he was asked to copy the same cross with his clever right hand, he could not. He drew several lines incoherently, as though he could only see small segments of the cross at a time, and he could not finish the model. With six separate strokes, he managed to draw only half of the cross. Prompted to do more, he added a few lines but then stopped before completing it and deemed it finished. It was clear that this was not due to lack of motor control, but instead there was a defect in the concept. There was a striking contrast to the quick understanding of his mute half. What had Gazzaniga discovered exactly?

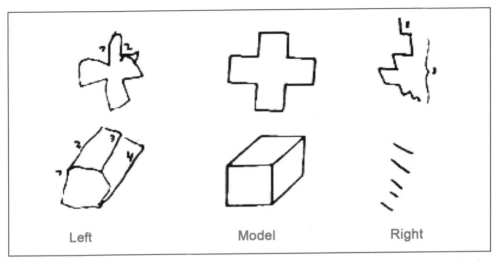

Left   Model   Right

Drawing by a person with a split brain. On the left side the right hemisphere's abilities to draw are clearly seen; however, on the right side the left hemisphere's inability to draw is evident.

■ Human brain anatomy

If we could look at a human brain we would see that it is divided into two identical halves, which consist of the same types of cells. However, evidence shows that they are very different: this is called functional lateralization. Each hemisphere seems to specialize in performing different tasks. Language is one of the most important tasks for human beings and in most people it is located in the left hemisphere. Research suggests that it is the center of activities related to speaking, reading, writing, logical thinking, and analyzing information. The right hemisphere specializes in controlling certain movements in synthesis, understanding, and communicating emotions.

"Activities related to logical thinking are in the left hemisphere and those related to synthesis and understanding are in the right hemisphere."

Initially, research was conducted with people who had surgically excised hemispheres. The hypotheses were criticized since they could not be tested on normal people. Thus alternative research was to be conducted on people who had not been intervened surgically. For this, sodium thiopental is sometimes used. This anesthetic is injected into the volunteer's neck, immobilizing half of his body for a short period of time. After about twenty seconds, the drug takes effect and psychologists have a few minutes to contact one of the hemispheres. When the right hemisphere is anesthetized, volunteers can recite letters, name days of the week, and repeat sentences. But when the left hemisphere is anesthetized, individuals have serious problems performing tasks related to speech.

Other studies, including positron emission tomography, also provide evidence for this lateralization. When people talk or calculate, they show great activity in the left hemisphere. But when they perform perceptual tasks, the activity of the right hemisphere increases.

■ I hear a voice inside me

At this point you may be wondering what all this has to do with mental diagrams. Have you asked yourself this question? Did you hear an inner voice? Do not panic, there is no elf inside your head that talks to you incessantly; it is your own voice.

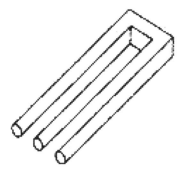

This is the famous devil's prong. While the right brain more or less accepts it, the left brain will be greatly upset by its lack of logic.

To be more precise, it is your left hemisphere's voice that uninterruptedly dialogues inside your head, and it is very difficult to silence it. This voice has a very specific purpose: to simplify the feelings and thoughts you have about the world around you. Yes, I know that sometimes this voice may be rude and judgmental, but remember it is a part of you . . . but not the whole.

THE BLIND AND THE ELEPHANT

There once was a town where all the inhabitants were blind. One day there came about a king and his retinue; he brought his army and encamped in the desert. The king had a huge elephant, which he used in battles and to instill fear in people. The villagers were eager to know about the elephant, and some of the blind in this community ran like crazy to get to know it. Since they ignored the shape or appearance of the elephant, they groped blindly to gather information by touching any part of its body. Each one thought he knew something because he could feel something.

When they returned to the city, its residents asked them about the shape and appearance of the elephant. The man whose hand had reached its ear said: "It's a large and extensive thing, rough and wide as a carpet." One who had touched the trunk said: "I can tell you how it really is. It's like a straight and hollow tube, horrible and destructive." One who had touched the hooves and legs, said: "It is strong and solid, like a column."

Each one had touched one part among many. All had erroneously perceived it. None of their minds knew it in its entirety: knowledge is not a companion to the blind.

> **"The two hemispheres are joined by the corpus callosum, a bundle of nerve fibers that connects the two sides."**

It may sound funny, but if we accept that we have an inner voice that constantly talks to us, it would be interesting to know to whom it speaks. Is there anyone else in there? Any discerning reader will notice that it is obviously talking to the right hemisphere. This is correct. In fact, the corpus callosum that unites the two hemispheres is a bundle of nerve fibers that keeps them connected. It is like a switchboard that sends and receives thousands and thousands of words per minute in both directions. However, there is one small problem: each hemisphere has its own language and sometimes communication is difficult. For example, if it is listening to a very drab and uninteresting speech the right hemisphere may get disconnected and start to fantasize and imagine other scenarios (like being at the beach sunbathing). At that moment, the left hemisphere was listening but hardly understanding any of the words. On the other hand, if you see paintings in a museum your right hemisphere will enjoy the landscapes and still life, but your left brain is bored, unable to intervene.

■ Two is better than one

The language of the left hemisphere is not the problem; it is the common language we use every day—words, phrases, and grammatical rules— that provide structure. We form phrases word by word and paragraphs phrase by phrase. In so doing, we combine phrases to form sentences

THOUGHTS WITHOUT THINKING

Zen meditation has been spreading worldwide for several years. The principle of this type of meditation is very simple; it is based on posture. All you have to do is sit without moving, and although it may not look like it, there is movement in everything. During the first minutes of meditation the mind is an open window through which a strong current of air blows: thoughts arise incessantly. Then, with increasing practice thoughts start to decrease and finally stop. When the wind stops blowing, the mind becomes a quiet place. Eliminating thought leads to a state of concentration called "shi" in Japanese. The kanji "shi" literally means to cease or to stop, and by this we mean that spiritual concentration brings tranquility.
However, this spiritual condition does not itself define true meditation. Simply stopping thoughts is merely one aspect of the true meaning of meditation and leads to a state of drowsiness called "kontin." The spirit cannot stay awake because that requires a certain amount of awareness and activity. This active monitoring is observation, "kan," the second component of meditation. "Shi" and "kan" together provide the correct meditative state of mind.

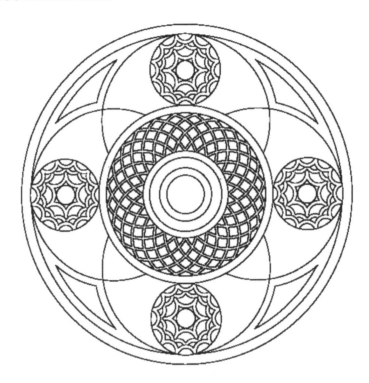

Eastern mystics have used mandalas for centuries in their meditations. Concentrate on the center of the pattern as you banish from your mind all other thoughts.

until we complete thoughts and ideas. This is the education we received: reading, speaking, writing, and reasoning. But what happens when we have to address new or complex material? And what if we have to make a difficult and personal decision? Usually we get lost in words when we are overwhelmed by large amounts of information we cannot process. That is when we get confused or when we start to overthink. That is when

RESEARCH PROCESS

When Tony Buzan began his inquiry on how he could use his brain more, he ran into the theory of the hemispheres. He investigated thoroughly and found that in it is the reason for our poor intellectual performance. He tried developing a technique to maximize the brain's potential 100 percent. That would mean a joint effort by each hemisphere: the left had to provide logic and classification, and the right had to provide creativity and a general overview. Words and images had to jointly play a single melody. Was this possible? The answer is yes.

the left hemisphere is going full speed trying to understand the problem and finding a solution, but understandably, the left hemisphere has its limitations. Sequential thinking is slow and it examines sections, but it has difficulty seeing the whole. Wouldn't it be wonderful to think simultaneously rather than sequentially, to be able to see the whole not just the parts? Well, you already posses that way of thinking; it just happens to be quiet and dormant. For a long time this manner of thought has been penalized, but now it is time for it to come out with greater force than ever. The right hemisphere is responsible for this kind of thinking; it uses holistic reasoning, and it is responsible for spatial thinking, visualization, and something that interests us a lot, creativity. Imagine for a moment that you had two brains instead of one. Wouldn't that be amazing?

CONCENTRATION TEST

Inside you there may be two minds that represent different entities. Surely they are not always in agreement. Have you ever had to try to convince yourself through logical justifications? Apparently, the speaker tries to convince the listener. To learn more about these two elements we will do an experiment: our goal is to disengage the speaker (left hemisphere). Find a quiet and comfortable place, where nobody can bother you, and relax your body. Try to quiet down the constant internal conversation in your mind until it finally disappears. Let your mind go blank. Try it for two minutes.

Time is up. Did it fail? I am not surprised. Few people can do this exercise without having previously practiced yoga or another meditative technique. Now try it again, but while you concentrate repeat a special word over and over in silence. Find a word that is soft and pleasant, such as "buzz." Silently repeat it again and again; did you do better this time? This phenomenon is simple; by forcing the right hemisphere to perform a repetitive task with a word, it stays busy and thus we can connect with the right hemisphere.

RELAXATION EXERCISES

As you have seen, we are often caught up in tension and stress. To move forward on the path of holistic thinking we need a certain degree of inner calm, which is difficult to attain today. Here we suggest a relaxation technique that has been successfully used in hypnosis. And to keep the "speaker" under control we offer a few powerful techniques. Be aware that silencing the voice is a bit challenging, but if you practice the following exercises it will become a simple task.

👁 Exercise number 1: Countdown

Hypnosis has come a long way over the years. Currently, although there are many therapists who use it, is not yet well known how it works. We are interested in a helpful technique: like most relaxation techniques, it is based on distracting the left hemisphere while we access the right hemisphere, which can give us rest.

Look for a calm and quiet place and sit comfortably. Once your body is relaxed, close your eyes. From this point you have to work with both hemispheres; in this case you have to count down from sixty to one. While you silently count the number you also have to visualize it. You can imagine the numbers any way you want, but most importantly they should have great detail and colors. You have to see how they change every second:

60, 59, 58 . . .

When you reach 1 (if you get there) you will be in a great state of relaxation. Stay a few minutes in this state and then repeat the words "wake up, wake up" and then reincorporate easily.

◉   Exercise number 2: **The senate**

Sometimes it is almost impossible to stop listening to the left hemisphere. Sometimes it is very excited and it seems that nothing can stop it. For those times, use the technique of the senate. To do this you have to imagine that the inner voice you hear is a senate member's opinion. Imagine the voice of the senate telling you that you spoke too much in a debate. Then you have to allow a few minutes so that the voices of other senators, maybe not as loud, also express their opinions. Try to identify those speakers; surely you will be surprised.

◉   Exercise number 3: **Negative thoughts**

Maybe in your mind you hear a voice repeating negative thoughts over and over. It may tell you bad things, such as that you are useless or you will never amount to anything. Imagine for a moment that in your head there is a radio with switches. You can change the voice you hear, or you can make it slower or more distant. Another variation is to change the tuning of the radio and hear a friendly voice that encourages you through positive messages.

GOALS OF THIS CHAPTER

Rediscovering the world

The first basis for mental diagrams is acknowledging the existence of two distinct brain hemispheres. One of the main objectives of making mental diagrams is achieving the maximum degree of development of each one of them. Knowing and taking control of the two hemispheres is the basis of the mental diagrams technique.

The objectives of this chapter are:

- Recognizing the existence of two distinct hemispheres.
- Knowing the specific functions of each one.
- Applying relaxation and concentration techniques to develop mental diagrams.

3 Processes of the right hemisphere: The power of visualization

Every night we dream, even when we cannot remember our dreams. What is the purpose of dreaming? Why do we daydream? Can dreaming help us access mental diagrams? Throughout this chapter we will answer these questions and we will learn to talk with the right hemisphere through the process of visualization.

■ **The sleep study**

■ **The role of alpha thinking**

■ **The ring moves**

■ The sleep study

As the right hemisphere's functions were discovered, access to its full potential was achieved through dreams. Dreams have been and continue to be humanity's great enigma. Some authors claim that sleep is an evolutionary mechanism that encourages inactivity and that it is not specific to our species. As indicated in this theory, it is a way to keep still at night, as this was a dangerous time for our ancestors and, statistically, for us as well. However, most experts believe that sleep and dreams have much more important functions than one might suspect. One of these functions would be related to storing information. Through experiments, in which participants were awakened during stages of the deep sleep, it was verified that sleep was related to the storage and processing of information. Waking the subjects constantly demonstrated that they lost the ability to retain newly acquired information. Can we learn from dreams? Many experts say yes, but there is no need to fall asleep in order to learn; there are other ways.

■ The role of alpha thinking

Following research on dreams, it was found that there was a series of intermediate stages between waking and sleeping. These conditions were studied through encephalograms, and different types of brain waves were detected.

When we are awake and fully conscious our brain waves are at a relatively high frequency (14 to 30 Hz). They are called beta waves. As you get closer to a rest period, beta waves are replaced by alpha waves whose frequency is lower (8 to 13 Hz). And as you are falling asleep, delta waves appear, which are even slower.

"Dreaming is a state in which we emit alpha waves and in which the brain works at its full creative potential."

What was this research project's major finding? In moments of increased mental clarity and creativity we are in an alpha state. Apparently, we need moments in which we can get carried away into a dream state. When was the last time you had a dream? Can you see imaginary events or scenes while you are awake?

If so, I congratulate you. Although at school you were most likely discouraged to daydream, this ability has now become a powerful tool for you to maximize your brain's full potential. It is interesting to know what types of dreams are most common. To this end, a recent study was conducted and the most commonly reported dreams included:

- situations of success or failure.
- aggression or hostility (putting someone in their place).
- sexual or romantic fantasies.
- guilt (tortured by something that should have been said or done).
- solving a problem.

I suppose you have recognized your last dreams among one of these. What role do fantasies play? Psychology has not yet been able to give a clear and definitive response, but it offers some plausible hypotheses. On the one hand, it may be an escape from reality. For example, if you think that this text is not very interesting, you can manage to read these words, but your mind is elsewhere (I hope that is not the case). Another possibility is to alter your mood. If you imagine that you are going to spend a great weekend you are likely happier when you come to the end of your fantasy. And there are two other possibilities that I believe are more accurate—the first is based on finding solutions to current problems and the second is to provide behavior we want to set.

"The right hemisphere peaks in alpha state and is the natural language of images."

Indeed, sometimes when there is abundant data or a complicated problem, it is best to let the right hemisphere give us an overview of the subject. Has it ever happened to you that after going for a walk or stepping away you have found a solution to a complex problem you could not solve? That is because you parked your left hemisphere and allowed the right hemisphere to analyze the information comprehensively. Remember that our mute friend has the ability to organize information in new ways to find the best solution. The right hemisphere organizes information very quickly, but it does so through images. This type of holistic thinking is used in mental diagrams; to be able to use them you just have to learn its syntax.

■ The ring moves

If you want to know the power of dreaming and the right hemisphere, I suggest a simple experiment. To do this you need a gold ring and a 12-inch rope. Now tie the ring to the rope and hold the rope between your index finger and thumb.

Look carefully at the ring; you will see that it is impossible to prevent the pendulum from moving a little. Now imagine that the pendulum moves from side to side, and watch it carefully. What is happening? The pendulum is doing just that. Imagine now that the pendulum moves in a circle; focus, notice how it is changing. The pendulum goes round and round. What is happening? You might say "the power of the mind is directing the ring," which is true, but it is easier than you think. The language of the right hemisphere, by visualizing the ring in a straight line or in circles, unconsciously gave orders for the muscle to carry out this movement. Well, actually they were conscious orders, but visual language is a kind of language that we are not accustomed to, so we are amazed by it. I am not saying that we can move mountains with images, but if you learn to control the images you will be able to think creatively, solve problems, concentrate, and utilize mental diagrams fully.

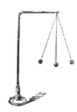

"The images that we visualize push us unconsciously toward action."

 ## VISUALIZATION TEST: **WHAT DID I EAT LAST NIGHT?**

Before exercising our visual brain we will perform a simple test to measure the extent to which you have developed your ability to visualize. I hope the result does not frighten you since this ability is more irregular than you can imagine. For example, some people visualize images in two dimensions, as if they were watching TV. However, others see the objects in three dimensions. Regardless of how you process visual information, we will try to estimate your current skill. Relax for a moment and visualize the scene from last night's dinner. Close your eyes and try to see all the details, the people, the atmosphere, the shape of the food, the flavor, the light, etc. You got it? Well, try to answer the following questions:

- Is it a clear or indistinct image?
- Are all the scenes defined with the same intensity or are some clearer than others?
- Is the picture in color or shades of gray?
- Were you able to see the entire dining room in a single image?
- Can you see the main course and focus the image clearly?
- Can you see everyone at dinner in detail?

Well, what are your answers? Were you able to respond with certainty or were there gaps in the images? If you had to score your answers, how would you rate?

1. I was present at dinner, but I do not remember anything.
2. I vaguely remember some things, but I cannot be sure of anything.
3. With much effort, I can re-create a good part of the dinner.
4. I accurately remember people, dishes, flavors, and even textures without difficulty.

If you scored a one or two, do not worry; most people have serious trouble remembering. The degree to which we can remember the details is very low, but it can be improved. The precision with which we can recall an object is closely related to the degree of our observation of the same, which indicates that we are not used to observing carefully. To bring images to life we have to put aside our verbal thinking and put some effort into using our unknown right hemisphere. How do we do that? Well, I suggest a series of exercises to strengthen your visual muscle, but you can start to train by asking yourself what it is that you actually see. Spend little moments of your life observing things around you. As you practice visualization, images will emerge naturally through the inexhaustible power of your right hemisphere.

👁 VISUALIZATION EXERCISES: LEVEL 1

Here I suggest two exercise levels to increase your visualization capability. This first level is simple and easy to perform. As you can see, they are more entertaining than it might seem.

👁 Exercise number 1: I have seen it several times

There are elements that are very familiar to us because we have seen them countless times, so it should be relatively easy to visualize them. If the images do not appear as sharp as you would like, do not worry; that is normal. To give them more life you have to first try to visualize their shapes, texture, colors, or sizes. First, focus on the shape and then on the details. You will see that the image slowly becomes sharper:

The face of a loved one

Your pet or a dog running

Your bedroom

An eagle in flight

Fluffy clouds

A childhood friend

A leafy oak

A beautiful sunset

A clear water spring

👁 Exercise number 2: I can imagine it

The mind can retain elements we have seen in real life, but it also has the ability to create the new and nonexistent; in this case they are mythological and dreamlike images. Close your eyes and try to visualize the following:

A unicorn

A fairy with butterfly wings

A giant ant

A choir of angels

A hippopotamus with a lion head

A river of chocolate

A talking giraffe

The Loch Ness monster

A phoenix

👁 Exercise number 3: The five images exercise

Many visual elements work by association. For example, thinking of a red sunset can make us think of an orange. We will see the importance of associations in mental diagrams, but for now we will use them to enhance our capabilities to visualize:

- Visualize five blue things (the sky, some flowers, a dress, etc.).
- Do the same exercise using red, yellow, and green.
- Visualize five things that are smaller than a finger (a pea, a marble, a clip, etc.).
- Visualize five things larger than a bus (a building, a blue whale, a plane, etc.).
- Visualize five living beings that can be found underneath the ground (a root, a worm, etc.).

👁 VISUALIZATION EXERCISES: LEVEL 2

As you have seen, the difficulty of the exercises in Level 1 was relatively low. I am guessing you had no trouble seeing the items and you did not have to make a lot of effort to concentrate. The following exercises are more abstract, but they are simple.

👁 Exercise number 4: TV Technician

In this exercise, visualize one of those old television sets with buttons that were manually tuned. Once you visualize it, tune in to a station with any image you like, such as a waterfall. At first you have to imagine it blurry, but as you move the dial to tune it, the image gets sharper. Use the buttons to modify the image and make it brighter, for instance. What happens when you change it? Visualize that the image becomes white and if you do the opposite, it darkens. The same can be done with the contrast, size, sharpness, etc. Try to completely control the images you see.

Sharpness	Brightness	Contrast
Size	Nuances	Color intensity

👁 Exercise number 5: **Feelings**

Now that we have complete control over the images, let us visualize positive feelings. Imagine a feeling like joy, trying not to recall a specific memory, but allowing the right hemisphere to show you its meaning of joy. To what extent can you vividly visualize this emotion?

Now try doing the same with the following emotions. Do not limit your imagination:

Hope	Love	Tenderness	Friendship
Satisfaction	Sympathy	Warmth	Excitement

👁 Exercise number 6: **Images of ideas**

This exercise is extremely important for mental diagrams. Later we will see that we need to be able to visualize the main idea. So we will practice creating images of ideas. For starters, try to create the image of Beauty. Do you see a specific image of something concrete, or is it an abstract

image of Beauty? Do you associate the idea of Beauty with certain
sounds, smells, tastes, or other sensations? Is it a big or a small idea?
Well, once you have found the notion of Beauty try the same with the
following ideas:

Change	Energy	Peace	Reality
Order	Harmony	Communication	Love

👁 Exercise number 7: **Brain Massage**

Now that you have a better grasp of your mental imagery you can create
your own relaxation exercises through images. Brain massages work very
well for me. As I massage myself, I start to feel revitalized and even get to
see the brain in better colors. Put it into practice and you will see results
from the start.

Visualize your brain inside your head. Imagine the space it takes up,
behind the eyes, on top of the spine.

Now, visualize that your fingers have the power to massage and soothe
away any tension. Start by giving a massage to the outer layer of your
brain, like when you wash your hair. Focus on the feeling of relaxation that
your fingers give you. Let all your tension vanish.

Allow this renewed energy, released by the massage, to flow into the
center of your brain. Allow those tangible, warm, and tingly sensations
to spread throughout. Give your brain a layered massage, starting with
the outer layer and progressively moving toward the center. If distracting

thoughts interfere, consider them as simple brain sensations. Visualize that you can massage any part of your brain and also massage away any distracting thought, as though you were cleaning. Afterward limit yourself to experiencing the feeling of inner relaxation. Do nothing but remain seated, enjoying your present state.

GOALS OF THIS CHAPTER

The power of visualization

To create mental diagrams it is essential to work with visual images. The starting point stems from what we call the central image. It is therefore very important that you acquire enough skill to be able to visualize without problems.

The objectives of this chapter are:

- Unlocking the enormous potential of the right hemisphere
- Understanding the importance of daydreaming as a doorway to alpha thinking
- Getting good mental relaxation through daydreams
- Beginning to cultivate extraordinary visualization powers used by great geniuses

4 Processes of the right hemisphere: Rediscovering the world

Now that we have begun to awaken the right hemisphere, can we get to know its hidden potential? What is the brain's storage capacity? Why are images so important in advertising? Can we present visual information through drawings? This chapter will cover these issues and you will learn how to make basic drawings and sketches to process and store visual information.

■ **Thousands of images per minute**

■ **The imaging industry**

■ **The right hemisphere can also draw**

■ Thousands of images per minute

Have you ever wondered why certain scents remind you of long-forgotten scenes? Why is it that the shower feels scorching hot at first and then it is at the right temperature? Why does the moon seem larger when it is on the horizon than when it is above? If you have ever been curious about these type of issues, you have unwittingly ventured into the amazing world of perceptions. In fact this topic is not new, and it is one of the oldest fields of study within psychology. Over many years and many experiments, research has yielded an interesting result: our senses are much more developed than

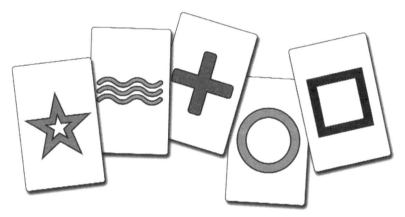

Through Zener cards, there have been attempts at investigating alleged divination capabilities through a scientific method.

we might suppose. For example, would you bet (a dollar, for instance) that you would be able to notice a teaspoon of sugar dissolved in 7.5 liters of water? You better not bet, because you would lose. Our senses are receptive and they have a direct connection with the brain. The existence of a sixth sense has long been speculated. Some psychologists have been interested in the existence and meaning of extrasensory perception.

All types of research studies have been conducted and the results have been rather poor and inconclusive. Some of the research suggests that people who demonstrate this powerful perception are in fact very sensitive. Almost unconsciously they are able to capture and interpret glances, gestures, sounds, and smells. If we add to this a good ability to think with the right hemisphere (through images) we get a clairvoyant! I hope this does not frighten you; this is not a book about developing your extrasensory powers, although that may seem like a possible side effect if you work with mental diagrams.

You may have noticed that of all the senses, the most important is vision. In fact, this is not surprising since we are surrounded by light, that wonderful energy that drives our weak planet's life. Actually, for most of us, our vision is the most important means of obtaining information from the world. It is so important that we have a specialized hemisphere just for capturing and processing visual stimuli. But what limits are there in our visual perception? Can it be part of the key to our data super-processor? It seems so. In the '70s there were a series of experiments that sought the limitations of our visual abilities of perception, retention, and recall. One of the best-known experiments was that of the 2,560 slides. The slides were shown to all participants with a duration of one second per slide. Then, the participants had to find the slides within a set of 5,120 images, among which half of them were previously exposed. The result was that the participants accurately recognized and matched between 85 and 95 percent of the slides. The most striking fact about this experiment is the amazing image processing power of our right brain (and its breakneck speed). In fact, the researchers predicted that even if the number of slides increased to 25,000 the results of the experiment would have bean similar!

> **"The right hemisphere can process thousands of images at breakneck speed."**

■ The imaging industry

There is no doubt that the phrase "a picture is worth a thousand words" is absolutely true. Images stimulate a wide range of cortical skills: colors, shapes, lines, and dimensions feed the right hemisphere. The evocative power of images is essential to create associations and strengthen creative thinking and memory. The advertising industry knows the power of images and takes advantage of them to seduce the brain's silent half through associated emotions.

> **"You can communicate with the right hemisphere through pictures."**

An interesting derivation of this power is in logos. Something as simple as a small design can cost millions of dollars; how is that possible? Through advertising the logo is associated with a range of emotions that represents the product or service. Experts say that the best logos are those that are easy to read, speak for themselves about the product, and need no explanation. Our aim is for you to be able to make a good drawing because in order to create mental diagrams you need this ability.

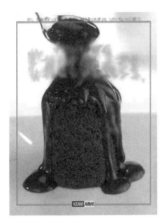 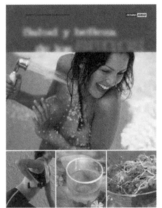 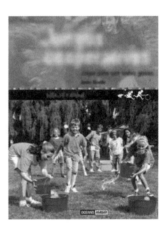

Have you any idea of the contents of these books just by glancing at them?

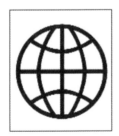 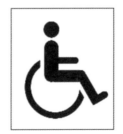  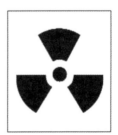

Try to guess what these icons refer to; see how you recognize them at a glance.

■ The right hemisphere can also draw

One of the first contacts I had with the theory of the hemispheres was not through psychology but through drawing. When I was young I had artistic interests, so to speak, and among them was drawing. In my efforts to learn the secrets of this noble art I read a lot of books on "learning to draw." However, my results were not correlated to the large amount of books I read, so becoming a Leonardo da Vinci was difficult. When I was about to abandon my aspirations I came across a book entitled *Drawing the Right Side of the Brain*, by Betty Edwards. In it was the following question: Why is it that adults draw so poorly? You may think that good artists have a gift, a natural talent that makes them exceptional art beings. All other beings, myself included, do not have that talent, so they can make zero contributions to the arts. However, Betty's answer was different: she said that our learning process for drawing had stopped at school age. At some point, drawings begin to be seen as childish and useless, while other things such as physics, mathematics, or chemistry come to be regarded as "serious." If you do not think this statement is correct, do a little test: draw a simple item like a car. You probably started by drawing a pair of wheels, then you made the outline of the car, and with a little luck you have drawn windows and headlights, all in two dimensions. Do you think this is the most that millions of neurons in your brain can do? Well, the result is a bit poor. What happened exactly? The answer is simple, this car was drawn . . . by your left hemisphere! Yes, the one that is logical,

RESEARCH PROCESS: CONSCIENCE

There is a whole series of investigations suggesting that each hemisphere has its own conscience, even its own values. More than one author has come to regard the conflicts with which we sometimes struggle as though there were two parts to each of us, one more logical and the other more emotional. An interesting experiment proceeded to learn the limits of the possible struggle between the left hemisphere (the talker) and the right hemisphere (the mute). A volunteer with a high level of development in the right hemisphere was given a simple test. He was given words and he had to classify them as good or bad. The two hemispheres regarded some words equally, but other words like "mother" or "sex" were classified as good by the left hemisphere and as bad by the right hemisphere. This indicates that each hemisphere may have its own system for assigning values to people and things. In a separate trial he was asked what he wanted to be when he got older, and while the left hemisphere said "architect," the right hemisphere said "racecar driver." If you are unconvinced by what I say then do a simple test. The next time you have trouble getting out of bed to go to work, listen to your inner voice for a moment. The left hemisphere may be reminding you about the importance of getting up to meet your obligations, while the right hemisphere is enjoying your dream state and trying to persuade you to keep from moving. Right?

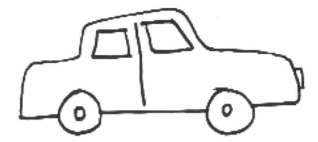

Car drawn by a thirty-four-year-old adult

analytical, and sequential. What your left hemisphere did was to translate the concept of a car to its most basic forms.

Usually, if you repeat this exercise with other objects such as a tree or a house, the results are similar. As you can see, they are representations without details, without life, extremely lacking. The right hemisphere is responsible for our artistic skills, but having been silenced for years, it cannot express itself.

"To learn to draw we have to let the right hemisphere take control."

Betty Edwards, with the advice of Nobel laureate Roger W. Sperry, first developed a practical application of the new theory of lateral thinking. According to her explanation, our culture rewards the left hemisphere's dominance and pushes away the right hemisphere to the point where the left even takes over tasks that do not belong to it, such as drawing.

Learning to draw is not a matter of innate gifts (although obviously having them does help), but instead it is about letting the right brain take control. Why is it so important to learn to draw to be able to make mental diagrams? For the simple reason that imagery is the natural language of the right hemisphere, and we need to learn to relate to it by using its language.

I guess you are not yet ready for a crash course in drawing, but do not be scared; I prepared it in such a way that you will find it easy.

👁 QUICK DRAWING "COURSE"

The objective of learning to draw is to discover your own personal expression and feelings through your strokes. Contrary to what you might think, making a drawing, diagram, or sketch is a work of experimentation and communication. Some people focus their drawings almost in a mathematical and realistic way, while others do it freely and subjectively. Regardless of the method, the fact is you have to find your own expression, your own trademark. Part of the secret is to discover what you want to express and convey that feeling using a pencil.

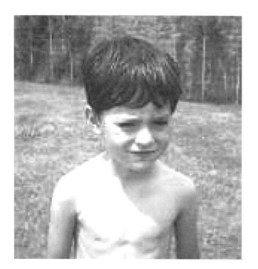 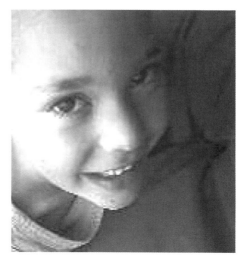

The photo on the left has little dimension and appears flat, while the one on the right has a strong three-dimensional effect. Which one do you think is more personal?

The first step in learning this new language is through observation. You must relearn to see information with renewed sight and translate that to paper. Imagine that this is a new language that you did not previously know. Most people speak their native languages fluently (I hope you are one of them) and build sentences according to rules and structures. However, when you learn a second language, you start from scratch and have to acquire extensive knowledge about the pronunciation, structure, and rules of that language. Something similar happens in this new language of the right hemisphere, the visual language. But do not worry;

it is easier and more fun than learning English. Furthermore, we will focus only on the most important point: the shapes.

"We must learn to see again, but differently."

Observation and lines

If you look carefully at any object, you will see an amazing combination of textures and tones. Light sheds on objects allowing us to discover its forms. The same object changes completely depending on the light it receives. Have you ever noticed how you perceive the photos you take of your family and friends? Upon observation they may look flat and lifeless. You are left with the impression that you could not capture the moment, emotion, or personality in the photograph. This is because whoever took the picture "does not know how to see." Professional photographers have learned to see with different eyes and their photos show a good range of tones, and depth, and furthermore, they explore the composition from new angles. In doing so, they manage to get photos with personality. I will not ask you for all that; our basic drawing course is much simpler.

  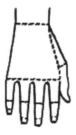 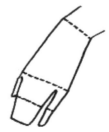

The only thing we will do is experiment with form. Initially, think that in nature there are no such things as lines; they are an abstraction. Although they do not exist, they are very useful for us to represent the objects we observe. Any element can be broken into lines. The secret to drawing is in describing the item through basic and simple lines. Many people believe they lack the ability to mimic forms, but this is incorrect. If you have an average ability to write then you are already a designer. The elements are composed of lines and basic geometric shapes, such as circles, squares, rectangles, etc. Making a circle or a straight line may seem like a difficult task, but they are familiar shapes. Do you want to see? Just draw an uppercase "O." There, you already have a perfect circle.

And now draw an uppercase "I." There you have a straight line. Through writing we are used to drawing strokes, some of them very complex. Use the shapes of the letters to sketch and draw elements. As you can see, there is a large collection of resources for you to begin making works of art.

Exercise number 1: Simple shapes

The first exercise is to break down the figures into simple geometric elements: circles, lines, triangles, squares, rectangles, etc. All you have to do is trace the shape over the picture and then repeat these figures in the box next to it. As you will see in the example, this is a simple and fun exercise.

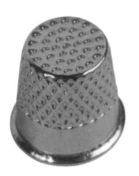 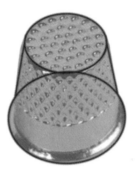 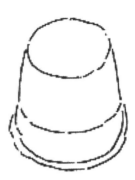

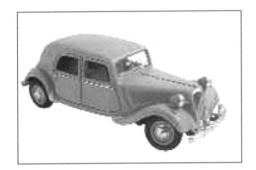 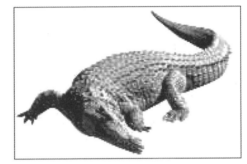

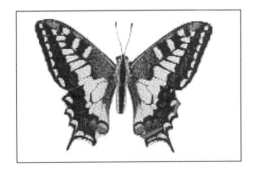 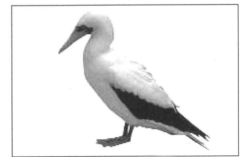

You are surely bound to like this exercise, so I suggest you practice with old newspapers and magazines. Look for those images that you like most and trace their basic geometric shapes over them. You will discover nature's architecture while helping the planet recycle paper in a useful way.

Exercise number 2: Your identity

A good way to know yourself is through your belongings. There are many things that represent you and which you know very well. You may be proud of your home, your plants, or your car. What better way of capturing them for posterity through your new skills! However, I must warn you that this exercise has an added challenge. In the previous exercise you looked at the basic shapes of two-dimensional pictures, which made it easy. In this case you have to make a life drawing, and this means that you must find three-dimensional geometric shapes. If you do not get it right the first time do not get discouraged; it is a matter of a little practice. Are you ready? Well, make a list of five items that represent your personality. These elements can be objects, animals, clothes, gear, etc.

Exercise number 3: The human figure

In most mental diagrams there are always human figures. It should come as no surprise given that people are some of the most important elements in our lives. Learning to draw the human figure with emotions is one of the most important parts of learning this technique. Here I give you a series of photographs that have to be broken down into their simple forms. Once you have made a sketch, try to add details to give it character; try to trace their personalities.

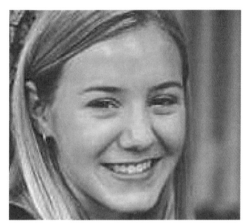
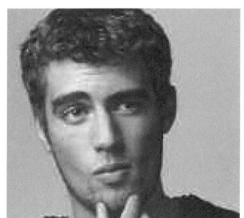
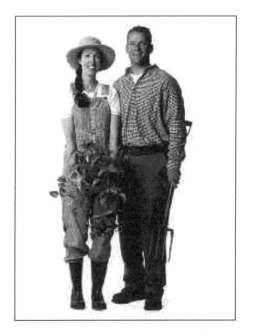
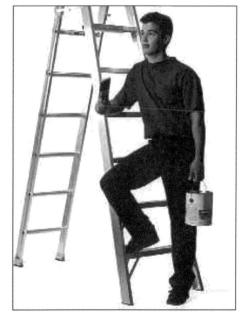

Exercise number 4: **Your objectives**

Now that you are an expert, we can go on to the representation of concepts. This time I will ask you to do an exercise that is very close to doing mental diagrams; you will illustrate your objectives using visual language. Imagine that you are studying and your goal is to pass—what would this look like? Are you willing to try? Think of three objectives you have set for yourself and draw them.

GOALS OF THIS CHAPTER

Rediscovering the world

Mental diagrams are powerful in part because they work with visual information. The brain's ability to process this information is almost unlimited. Images evoke strong associations, this triggers the creative process, and memory is strengthened. Learning to draw is essential to using the mental diagrams technique.

The objectives of this chapter are:

- Strengthening storage capabilities and memory recall using imagery.
- Stop resisting the use of images in learning.
- Increasing the aesthetic pleasure, that is, to enjoy the images themselves.
- Start thinking of drawing as one of the keys to creating mental diagrams.

---

5 Processes of the left hemisphere: The universe of words

It is commonly believed that good use of language is linked to high levels of intelligence, but is that true? Do writers (like me) denote some kind of intelligence? Where is the limit to words? Do words condition our thoughts?

This chapter will address these issues and we will train our left hemisphere in the use of language.

- **Word release**

- **A hundred thousand entries**

- **I have no words to express it**

- **Do we think what we say or say what we think?**

■ Word release

So far we have spent much of this precious book liberating the right hemisphere of its silence, but we must also pay attention to releasing the left hemisphere. You might have been under the impression that the left hemisphere has nothing to say and a lot to be quiet about. That is partly correct and partly incorrect. Our chatty hemisphere has the power of language, an ability that is so important that it makes us a unique species.

To get an idea of its importance, just consider that evolutionarily we developed an entire hemisphere solely for this function. Also, it is not just words that dominate this hemisphere but also the logic to articulate them and the rules governing their composition. Later we will see the great importance of the speaking hemisphere's capabilities for the development of mental diagrams, but for now remember that it is related to words and logic.

■ A hundred thousand entries

Today, most scientists say the only thing that separates us from other species is the use of language. This does not mean that other species do not communicate. From bees with their extraordinary dance to indicate the direction and distance of pollen to complex sounds made by whales traversing miles across the ocean, almost all animals exchange information.

However, the richness and complexity with which the human species does it far exceeds any other species known so far, at least among those known on planet Earth. We could define our language as a system of symbols with rules that are used to transmit information. How much information do you think you could pass along? An estimate tells us the answer is a lot, in fact, an almost unlimited amount. Currently there are a hundred thousand entries in the dictionary and the numbers of possible combinations between them are almost infinite. Is intelligence related to the ability to use words? Apparently so, and since the beginning of psychology it has been used as a "predictor" of school performance. Even in early intelligence studies, correlations were found between language use and intelligence level. This is not too strange, since we have to remember the importance of logic in language. This logic is present through syntax, which is defined as the rules by which words can be combined to create meaning. To see the difference between the meaning of words and their logical rules, read the following sentence:

"Purple ideas eat furiously."

If you look closely, you will notice that this sentence is grammatically well constructed, but it has no meaning. Rather, the phrase is well built and the words carry meaning, but they make no sense.

In an experiment to see the scope of the rules, dolphins were taught a series of words with their syntactic rules. The dolphins responded to commands given by their observers; these orders were simple: "bring the ball," "do a flip," etc. Once the dolphins had learned them, they were given orders using incorrect grammar to see what they did. One possibility was that the dolphins tried them without success, but contrary to expectation, the dolphins ignored the poorly constructed orders because for them they had no logic.

> **"Language is built on words, their meanings, and the logical rules that structure them."**

■ I have no words to express it

Has it ever happened to you that you want to communicate an idea or a feeling and you cannot find the right words? It seems incredible that among over one hundred thousand words you cannot find the right one to express yourself. This sometimes happens because there are sensations that are difficult to experience clearly and logically. We often process information visually through the right hemisphere and we see the ideas clearly, but when we try to explain them in words they lose their power and meaning. It is in those moments when we say, "No words can express what I feel." I recently signed up at a gym to stay in shape. The truth is that I have a sedentary life, so I decided to do something about it. Do you know how I felt the day after the first training session? You could say that my bones, muscles, joints—in short, everything—ached, but you may have noticed that with a formal description I am unable to convey my true feelings.

How about if I tell you that I looked as though "a pack of wild horses had run me over"? I guess now you can perfectly understand how I felt.

Poets know our language limitations and therefore look for new ways to alter it in order to transmit their feelings exactly. As a result, some linguists distinguish what they call surface structure and deep structure. The surface structure refers to the actual words people use and what is evident in them; however, the deep structure refers to information that underlies those words and gives it meaning.

■ Do we think what we say or say what we think?

For a long time psychologists asked themselves the following question: To what extent does language influence our perception of reality? A line of study is based on the fact that language conditions the way we perceive things. From this point of view, people of different countries perceive the world differently, because their thinking is conditioned by the words available to them. For example, Eskimos have many ways to describe snow, so they view it with greater regard than we do because in English there is only one word for "snow." Imagine a more disturbing example. Think of a person living in a society that has a wide range of words for weapons—what kind of ideas will this person have of the world? If we apply the same logic, this person will think that the world is a violent place. By contrast, other researchers claim that our thoughts condition our words.

In another experiment, a parrot named Alex was taught some words and their meanings. He was taught over eighty objects and facts and he learned to ask for things he wanted, such as "I want to bathe." When Alex first tasted an apple he called it "banerry" and he clung to this word even though they tried to teach him to say "apple." The explanation for the phenomenon is that the apple looked like a cherry but it tasted like a banana, so the parrot created the most logical new word to designate the new fruit: "banerry."

> **"We must increase our vocabulary to better understand the world."**

Have psychologists been able to answer the riddle about whether we are conditioned by our vocabulary? To be honest, this enigma remains unclear. For example, the fact that a culture has few words for weapons does not mean it cannot differentiate or create new words to designate them, as did Alex. For a tribe in New Guinea there are only two colors in their vocabulary; one of them refers to bright and warm and the other refers to dark and cold. Does this mean that they fail to see other colors? In research, it has been observed that they recognize other colors, but in their context they do not need these words. But what is certain is that we do not live in New Guinea and to express ourselves in our society we need plenty of words, so the more vocabulary you possess and the better you articulate its logic, the more resources you will have to express your ideas. And the benefits do not stop there; you also acquire a direct training on your logic. But you are not alone. You have an entire hemisphere waiting to be developed—we are talking about the left hemisphere. Here I suggest a series of practical exercises that are essential to strengthening the left hemisphere and will allow you to master mental diagrams.

EXERCISES TO STRENGTHEN THE LEFT HEMISPHERE

Below, I describe a series of exercises in which you will be able to train using words. These exercises are to be done with a partner, so they are a good way to spend an afternoon using the skills of your speaking hemisphere. Relax and enjoy!

Exercise number 1: An improvised speech

I give you a series of words for which you have to say four related phrases aloud. Try to make rich and meaningful sentences. Are you ready? Go!

Sugar	Camera	Money
Liquid	Sex	Grating
Bat	Key	Program
Absurd	Folder	Recording
Travel	Reality	Tiger
Sin	Home	Telephone

Exercise number 2: Synonyms

Finding synonyms for words is a good way to exercise your vocabulary, memory, and word meaning. Try saying as many synonyms as you can think of for the following words; you will see it is quite simple:

Sad	Important	Stubborn
Friend	Fearful	Funny
Attractive	Arrogant	Competent

Exercise number 3: **Every category**

Test your mind's ability to remember words in each category. If you want to make it more interesting, do it in alphabetical order. For example, for occupation you would have to say: architect, carpenter, janitor, etc.

Occupations	Cities	Musical instruments
Fruits	Animals	Countries
Articles of clothing	Tools	Sports
Books	Trees	Movies

Exercise number 4: **Descriptions**

There is no doubt that the ability to put into words all kinds of things and facts is essential. Do the following test and describe the following things to someone as though he or she was completely unaware of what these things are. Will he or she understand them?

Snow	Margarine
Sexual intercourse	A Bach fugue
Basketball	Your workplace
A sand castle	How to put on a jacket
Cleanliness	Cooking

Exercise number 5: New Words

Trying to make up words can be fun, but it is even more fun to make up their meanings. Try to describe in detail the meaning of the following words:

gropster	gurgitated	molished
chaintwist	zestpond	bruntle
plame	ebriate	beconic

GOALS OF THIS CHAPTER

The universe of words

Contrary to what you might think, mental diagrams also use words in their designs, but these words are carefully chosen and considered so that their meaning is most fitting to the idea you want to express. Learning, managing, and even creating new words is one of the skills that you must master when using mental diagrams.

The objectives of this chapter are:

- Paying more attention to the characteristics of words.
- Easily translating your thoughts into words.
- Reinforcing logic through your speech fluency.
- Increasing your vocabulary through synonyms.

6 Architecture of the brain: Idea association

Many psychologists compare the brain to a computer because both store and process large amounts of information, but how does the brain record information? How is it accessible? And how does the computer-brain theory fit in with the theory of the hemispheres?

This chapter will give answers to these questions and we will work on the brain's fundamental nature: its associative ability.

- **I cannot remember**

- **The most famous psychologist of the twentieth century**

- **Say whatever comes to mind**

- **What do apples taste like?**

- **The brain, a multiconnected computer**

■ I cannot remember

Film has frequently addressed topics related to psychology. I remember spending hours in front of a small black and white TV watching all kinds of movies, and that back then a movie, whether good or bad, was a big deal. However, even back then there were some movies I particularly liked—those were the ones with a psychological plotline. There is a particular film of which I have a special memory, and especially some key scenes. In one of these scenes, the protagonist, Gregory Peck, had a dream. In this dream he sees himself in front of black curtains full of watchful eyes. He pulls back the curtain and sees a man facing away from him. In the end the man turns around and it is himself. Do you recognize this film? It is *Spellbound* by Alfred Hitchcock, and the great artist Dali created this dreamlike scenery. Hitchcock was very interested in psychoanalysis, and many of his great films have strong psychological content. In *Spellbound* a young Gregory Peck has clear signs of amnesia and a strong sense of guilt. The female protagonist, a lovely Ingrid Bergman, realizes that whenever the young doctor sees parallel lines he becomes very tense and nervous and is not sure why. Apparently, the parallel lines are associated with some dramatic event in his life, but he does not know which one and cannot remember. The whole movie is based on discovering this dramatic association. But do not worry; I will not tell you what the association is, in case you have not seen this fascinating film.

"Our mind always makes associations, sometimes in unexpected ways."

■ The most famous psychologist of the twentieth century

Hitchcock's idea of the association to trauma was extracted from psychoanalytic theory. The famous Sigmund Freud, the father of psychoanalysis, always knew he wanted to be a historical figure, and boy did he achieve that goal. In a survey of the most influential men of the twentieth century, three key names appear: Marx, Einstein, and Freud. According to this study, a psychologist is one of the central figures of modern history. Not bad for this doctor who was ostracized by the scientific community for being a "degenerate." But what did he do for history to grant him such a predominant role? Well, he built a theory of personality disorders that revolutionized our present conception of human beings, which is no small feat. And what does this have to do with mental diagrams? If you are patient, you will soon see how he explored the association of ideas in depth.

■ Say whatever comes to mind

Freud investigated the human psyche through different means. One of the first methods he used was hypnosis. Through hypnosis he intended to give orders to make symptoms disappear, a goal he partially achieved. However, a strange phenomenon occurred in the middle of these sessions: patients spontaneously began to talk about events that had happened to them and which they did not remember consciously. Sometimes they linked one issue to another without any apparent connection, and most importantly, upon waking up they felt much better. Thus Freud began to use hypnosis as a gateway to recover lost healing memories. But new problems arose: one of them was that he had patients who were impossible to hypnotize. To overcome this setback, Freud had to work on other methods to access the unconscious.

Dreams are also a gateway to the unconscious

Between 1892 and 1896, Freud first uses the couch, the authentic seal of psychoanalysis. During this time he tries other methods to access the content; the new technique is to rest his hand on the patient's forehead while asking questions. With his hand on the forehead he asks the patient to free form the words *caretaker, robe, bed, car,* and *town* and thus the memories begin to emerge. "I was ten when my sister got sick and the caretaker took her into town in a car. I never saw her again." Freud discovered that words were linked. Sometimes these connections were unconscious and almost meaningless; however, they were bound by deep ties. Through this method he managed to reach the unconscious through a conscious state. Today psychoanalysis still uses the free association method to explore the lost corners of the mind. As indicated by the popular image, the patient lies on a couch in a semidark room. He cannot look at the analyst and the analyst does not look at him directly. That is when free association starts; this implies that anything that goes through the mind should be reported, no matter how trivial it may seem. Through this mental wandering, internal conflicts and hidden desires can be explored.

"**All words have dozens of connections, and in turn, each of these connections has dozens and dozens of new links.**"

■ What do apples taste like?

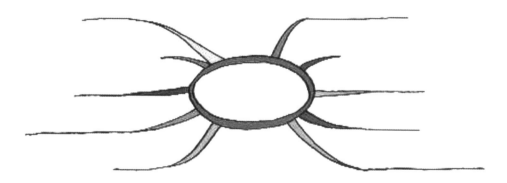

In our case we will not try to find internal conflicts hidden in the unconscious. Instead we will use the free association technique to create our mental diagrams. Let us do our own experiment using free association: imagine for a moment the taste of an apple, the fragrance of a flower, or the caress of a loved one. We can imagine the taste of an apple as the starting point that will take us to different elements and ideas. Think of the starting point as a main idea from which dozens of connections stem. It is similar to Internet links— sites that are in turn linked to new things that lead us to unknown places.

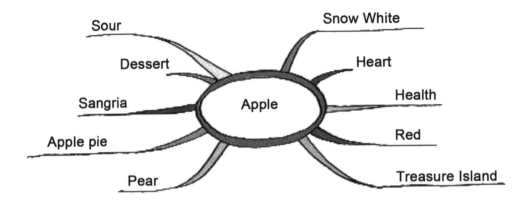

Similarly, as Freud discovered, thoughts are linked by association. Take the example of the flavor of an apple. I thought of a sour apple since I like those most. The first links that appeared are the dentist and a red apple. The red apple brings up Snow White's red apple and the sandy texture of red apples. If I follow the texture, it leads me to a sandy beach, where I have been wanting to go. And that idea is linked to the sea and the sun. When thinking about the sea, I think of jellyfish because the last time I went there were a lot of them. In this way, you could write dozens of books about associations and linkages that would fill entire libraries, and proof of what I say is in the works of Marcel Proust (which I like, by the way). I began this exercise by accessing the taste of an apple and I found myself among jellyfish. Isn't that amazing? Part of the explanation is that the brain works by processing associations, or in more technical terms, using connections.

A little experiment using the word *apple*. Each of the associated words could lead to dozens of associations, so with apple on one level we could easily reach one hundred words.

Each thought is formed by a specific network of connections. New thoughts create new connections, and apparently we have a few million of these precious cells. Some estimates have identified a few trillion possible connections, and that is a lot of links.

> **"Finding associations is also a creative method utilized by many artists."**

■ The brain, a multiconnected computer

Cybernetic theory helped shed some light on the mystery of processing. With the development of computers, psychologists came to compare the brain to a computer, and the two shared a number of similar processes. The key point of this comparison was that both are powerful data processors. Some characteristics shared by large data processors are:

1. Storing seemingly unlimited amounts of information for years and even decades.
2. Rewriting their own programs in response to new data entries and based on experience.

3. Simultaneously controlling a vast number of complex internal processes while handling external activities.

"Connections and associations allow us to store and retrieve thousands of memories."

But we are accustomed to using computers with keyboards, mice, monitors, and hard drives. So how does the brain's computer work? Very simply, through a system of associations and an information circuit that you create. The more associations you possess, the easier it will be to use your neuronal computer.

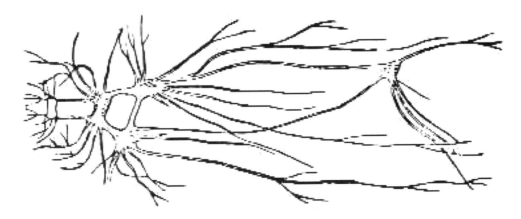

This is one of trillions of interconnected brain neurons that make up our special associative computer (a trillion is 1,000,000,000,000 units).

Now that you know each brain hemisphere's area of expertise and that the stored information is organized through associations, let us try to see how the two theories work together. Let us try a second experiment: imagine a loved one or friend. Close your eyes for a moment and think about this person. Did you do it? What did you see? Did you have a hard time trying to visualize? I guess not; after all the visualization practices we have done it must have been very simple. Usually, in a split second you will clearly see the concrete image of your friend. As you might guess, I made you exercise your right hemisphere in all its visual and holistic capacity. But you can also access your friend via your left hemisphere, although it may take a little longer. How? By asking yourself "What is this friend like?" You will give a verbal description in an orderly and consistent manner. Maybe you start by stating your friend's physical appearance, then you speak of his or her personality traits, interests, friends, work, etc., but you will always do it logically and sequentially because this task corresponds to the left hemisphere. As you can see, both hemispheres are prepared to make associations, each one with its own style.

👁 EXERCISES FOR FORMING ASSOCIATIONS

Now I suggest three simple exercises that will train you to form associations. For these exercises you need a pencil and a few coloring pencils so you can finally test your skills in the field of art (I will make you draw) and language (words and more words). If you are ready, take a deep breath and go.

HOW ASSOCIATIONS ARE FORMED

We have seen that associations can be created when two stimuli appear together, as it happened for Pavlov's dogs. Another way we create associations is by their resemblance. If we meet someone new, unconsciously the first thing we do is look for any similarities. The brain tries to map a stimulus, in this case the new person, by using already established neural structures, and in so doing, memories or people join together in our mind. Something similar happens to the protagonist of *Spellbound*. In this case, in his childhood a traumatic event occurs and it involves a fence that is perfectly outlined by vertical lines. And as an adult, whenever he sees parallel lines he always senses a tragic memory because the lines were forever associated with the painful event.

When we encounter a new stimulus, our brain also tries to find it, though it does not have a place for it yet. To do this, the brain recalls memories and preconceptions in order to associate similarity. For example, when the United States of America was colonized, Native Americans had never known a train before. As soon as they saw a train, they looked for associations; in this case they called it "iron" because of the material from which it was built (first association) and "horse" because it moved fast (second association). They took two familiar concepts and associated them with a new concept.

RESEARCH PROCESS: PAVLOV'S DOGS

Often, discoveries are not the result of hard research, as we tend to think, but rather the result of chance or an unforeseen observation.

This is what happened to Ivan Mestrovic Pavlov, the Russian scientist who discovered conditioning. Initially, Pavlov researched the digestive process in dogs. During his work he noticed a curious fact: all the dogs began to salivate upon seeing food, even minutes before tasting it. Some dogs even drooled simply by hearing the footsteps of people who normally fed them. The dogs had learned food signals and had associated these signals to the act of eating. From these observations, Pavlov investigated how associations are formed, and in a classic experiment he succeeded in associating the sound of a bell to eating.

Sometimes associations are created when events occur simultaneously. For example, I am sure that when you smell popcorn you think of the movies. How was this association created? By eating popcorn every time you are at the movies.

◐ Exercise number 1: The liquid element

Now you will perform a simple exercise of word association. Set aside the center space for the keyword, which is water. Find ten associations, however wild and crazy they may seem; do not try to find their meaning.

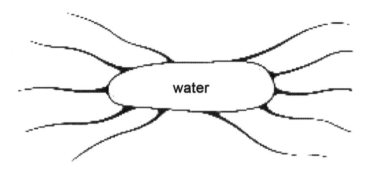

Once you complete the exercise, and if you dare, continue to add associations to those words.

◉   Exercise number 2: Home, sweet home

Now that you are an expert at creating word associations, I am going
to ask you to do a similar exercise, but visually. You will create visual
associations through pictures, following the same previous diagram. In
this case you have to create associations with the concept of home. To
help you, here is my own diagram for the word "home." If you have trouble
finding associations, remember alpha thinking; allow yourself to daydream
and visualize.

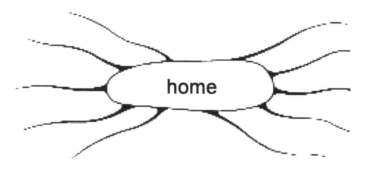

Exercise number 3: Alaska

This is the third associations exercise. In this case we will find things associated to the word *Alaska*. This time, you must also make ten associations, but here you can use words and pictures, or a combination of both. For each association draw a line that links the Alaska diagram to each word or picture you add. How did it turn out?

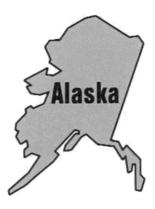

GOALS OF THIS CHAPTER

The association of ideas

Mental diagrams work with images, words, and associations. Associations provide the ability to discover the richness of thought and explore the enormous creativity in it. They also help memory by creating associative routes. Association is the third essential element for creating mental diagrams.

The objectives of this chapter are:

- Understand how associations work to process information.
- Increase the number of brain connections by means of free association of ideas.
- Use associations as a creative method.
- Learn to use associations through pictures and words.

7 Naturalistic intelligence: Classifications

I do not know if you ever collected music albums, stamps, videos, books, posters, butterflies, etc. Have you ever wondered why we have a tendency to seek, collect, and accumulate objects? Why do we always look for methods to classify and sort them? Do you like insects? Is this a useful ability?

This chapter will reveal the purpose of our naturalistic intelligence and we will do some practical exercises on order and classification.

- **Too much music**

- **It is harmless and edible**

- **Naturalistic intelligence**

- **Charles Darwin**

■ Too much music

How many music CDs do you have? If you are not a music fan you may only have a dozen, if you like it in moderation you may have a hundred, and if you really like it you may have over 500 discs.

At first, I had a small space reserved for them, but as the collection grew, I kept having to extend the shelf. There was an additional problem: What criteria should I use to classify the music? With so many discs I started having serious problems finding the music I wanted.

At first I thought of doing a standard classification—that is to say sorting it by type of music: classical, "new age," and international pop—but this system soon proved to be very limited.

In view of the complexity of this problem, I decided to gather all the discs and group them by similarities. There were new categories that I had not previously considered, such as music from India, of which I had about ten albums, or some bands that had a right to their own space because of their many albums in my collection.

But does sorting have anything at all to do with mental diagrams? The answer is yes, a lot. Under this chapter of "classifications" we will now find the latest concept we need to create and to design our own mental diagrams: order.

■ It is harmless and edible

Man has always been surrounded by endless amounts of complex information. This wealth of information, coupled with man's innate curiosity, produces an explosive cocktail. How can humans understand so much information? Well, it has its own support tools. Imagine for a moment that you are a prehistoric man, before writing came about. Accumulating information and knowledge was essential for your survival, and this information was partly transmitted from father to son, so you were like a walking encyclopedia. For example, knowledge about the animals that roamed the jungle was very important, so it was necessary to know if they were:

- harmless or dangerous
- edible or inedible

It may seem like a very basic classification, but back then it was of vital importance. In fact, classification was more complex; they also had to know if the animals were alone or in packs, if they could use their pelts, if they could be easily transported, etc.

Something as seemingly simple as recognizing an animal is much more complex than you might imagine. Think for a moment about the concept of "insect." Within this designation there are two complex and powerful mental processes. The first is that all insects have a resemblance and they have something in common. Clearly, you have unconsciously internalized this similarity, so it can be hard to explain the characteristics they share. The second process is to know the differences among them to discern which are insects and which are not. A simple example is that you could assume that insects are small, but what is small? There are insects that measure up to a foot. The world's largest roach, a native of Australia, is as big as the palm of your hand. If we go back to another era, some ancient cockroaches measured six feet; one was a centipede called "Arthorepleura." You see, something as simple as its size is already questionable. Putting the giant cockroaches aside and moving on, what is clear is that man, or rather the human mind, seems to depend heavily on the recognition of common groups, particularly collections of objects that we call grouping. Apparently, the left hemisphere is responsible for this function of recognition because it creates categories and provides them with a logical working name.

> **"The process of sorting involves finding similarities among some elements and their differences from other elements."**

■ Naturalistic intelligence

Howard Gardner, an eminent developmental psychologist, developed the theory of multiple intelligences. According to this theory, intelligence is a specialized adaptive process. Innovation is based on the assumption that we do not have a single intelligence; instead we have different types of intelligences with varying degrees of development. Thus there may be a person with a high mathematical intelligence, but with zero musical intelligence. There is one of these intelligences we want to emphasize; it is called naturalistic intelligence. According to Gardner, this intelligence was born through evolutionary steps, as the survival of an organism depends largely on its ability to differentiate similar species. With this understanding we could avoid our dangerous predators and seek our food. Accordingly, we can agree that there are other species that have this intelligence, but our species has developed it extraordinarily. Gardner defines the naturalist as someone who is skilled in recognizing and classifying the numerous species (flora and fauna) in its environment. This sounds pretty good, but a few things have changed from our prehistoric times until today. Does this intelligence remain valid in our time? Sure. A child can easily distinguish plants, birds, or dinosaurs, but thanks to this sorting capacity, he or she can also distinguish brands of athletic shoes, cars, marbles, or soccer teams. Clear evidence of its origin lies in children's strong interest in animals and plants, not to mention dinosaurs. I remember when my little son discovered the world of these large lizards: that was a revelation for him. We had to give him all kinds of explanations, read books, watch movies, and even buy figurines of these prehistoric animals (miniatures, of course). In this case, my son made his own dinosaur classification. The first classification was based on whether they could fly, live in water, or live on land. The second category, applicable only to the terrestrial type, was intended to find whether they ate meat or plants. For him this second point was the key to figuring out their degree of aggressiveness.

> **"The naturalistic intelligence is essential for categorizing ideas, concepts, and other items."**

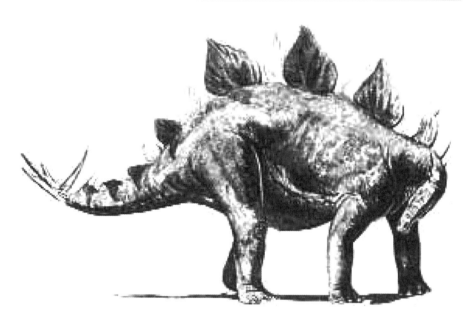

Since I am already an expert on dinosaurs, I give you the following riddle: Based on your experience, and using your common sense, is this prehistoric animal, called a stegosaurus, a carnivore or a herbivore?

[Answer: it is a herbivore for two reasons, the first being that it has developed defensive plates instead of attack features, and second, that his jaw is not as big and strong as that of carnivores.]

▪ Charles Darwin

There is no doubt that we all have the ability to classify objects, events, and people with high precision. This is partly because we have been programmed to perform such functions. But there are people in history who have excelled because they possess a well-developed faculty; in this case Charles Darwin is a good example of naturalistic intelligence.

As a child, Darwin seems to have been more of a dreamer than a child prodigy. He enjoyed long walks alone and from his earliest youth he was a passionate lover of nature. As he said, "I was born a naturalist." Every aspect of nature aroused in him a great curiosity. He was considered an ordinary child, or rather slow compared to the average. It was said that he was very slow to learn, and once his father rebuked him saying, "You will never amount to anything, all you care about is hunting, dogs, and killing rats, you will become an embarrassment to yourself and your family." Indeed, he preferred to collect animals, shells, eggs, vegetables, and minerals, as well as read books about nature above all other activities. Despite the bad omens that his father, peers, and teachers foretold, Darwin did very well in the natural sciences. Before Darwin's time scientific classifications of living things already existed. The science of classification is called taxonomy. This word is composed of two others: "taxis," which is order, and "nomo," science.

Before Darwin made his appearance, there was a clear and useful classification of living things, but it was the young Charles who could give a reason for the existence of these groups. Charles Darwin stated unequivocally that the members of a taxon (group) are similar because they are descended from a common ancestor.

For example, the similarities between a zebra and a horse are due to the fact that they share a common ancestor. Applying the same idea to the human species created a controversy that continues to be disputed even today.

As you may have already seen, we are all born with an innate sorting "kit." This capability, along with those mentioned previously, will be key to designing your mental diagrams. What if we start training this innate intelligence that sometimes remains hidden?

> **"Management and classification skills are key to designing mental diagrams."**

👁 EXERCISES FOR CREATING ASSOCIATIONS

The following exercises are prepared to help you exercise your sorting skills. Relax and let the left hemisphere take control freely. I bet you will find them very interesting.

👁 Exercise number 1: **The shopping list**

Here is a simple exercise to do with the shopping list. You have to group different products so that when you go to the supermarket it will be easy to find them in each section.

Tea	Detergent	Bicycle	Cookbook
Cushion	Coffee	Sugar	Chicken
Soda	Diapers	T-shirt	Ballpoint pen
Bread	Paper	Batteries	CDs
Tuna	Potatoes	Peanuts	Butter
Oil	Milk	Tomatoes	Eggs

👁 Exercise number 2: **Positive attitudes**

You will notice that the previous exercise was very easy. This one will be a little more difficult; you have to make new classifications, but in this case using a list of positive attitudes that would be good to have (or at least consider having).

This sounds easy, but it is rather complicated:

Joy	Self-confidence	Benevolence	Cooperation
Courage	Detachment	Determination	Discipline
Sweetness	Stability	Flexibility	Humility
Patience	Respect	Wisdom	Simplicity
Solidarity	Gentleness	Tolerance	Veracity

👁 Exercise number 3: **The naturalist's spirit (1)**

I am pretty sure you would like to emulate Darwin with his observations about nature's creatures. Well this is your chance to be a small ornithologist. Try finding an appropriate classification for the following birds and describe your criteria.

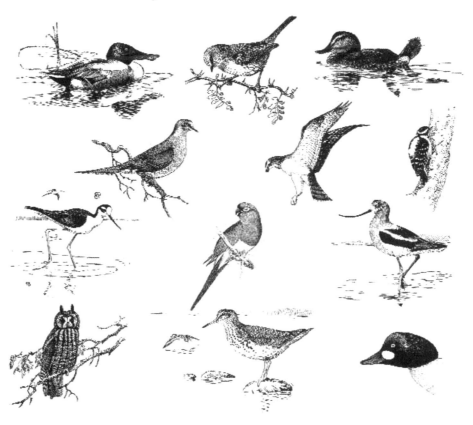

Exercise number 4: The naturalist's spirit (2)

Surely you are more eager to perform this type of exercise, so here I give you a second one. The first was of wildlife and this involves plant life. Group these trees by their similarity and describe the criteria you used.

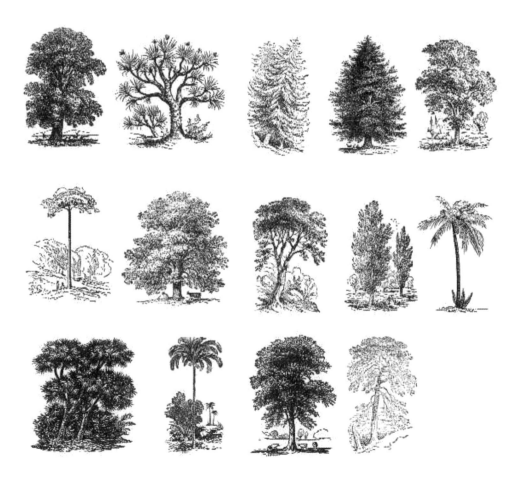

GOALS OF THIS CHAPTER

Classifications

Mental diagrams require a sorting capacity. As we shall see, at first we need to brainstorm ideas, words, images, and associations. But then we must give this brainstorm of ideas, words, and images some order and logical organization. The ability to classify ideas according to their similarity and the ability to create categories are essential to making mental diagrams.

The objectives of this chapter are:

- Understanding the key to the sorting process.
- Easily finding similarity criteria between items.
- Finding homogeneous groups and creating categories.
- Developing your naturalistic intelligence.

Integrating what has been learned

By now we understand how the brain works and we have developed the four basic skills needed to make mental diagrams.

In this second section we will define a mental diagram, know its process, and learn some rules to keep in mind.

The integration will be developed over two chapters:

- Ch. 8. In this section we will learn to create mental diagrams using four points: the central image, brainstorming, ordered structure, and other associations.

- Ch. 9. In this chapter we will see some rules that can help us have greater success with our mental diagrams.

8 Mental diagrams methodology: The orange

In this chapter we will define a mental diagram and we will construct one following step-by-step instructions. We will also see how to integrate everything that we have learned so far (hemispheres, associations, and classifications) within the mental diagram. Lastly, we will answer some remaining questions.

- **The mental diagrams recipe**

- **The central image**

- **Branched associations**

- **Ordered structures**

- **More associations and drawings**

- **Answered questions**

■ The mental diagrams recipe

Some time ago I read this saying: "The way to a man's heart is through his stomach." I meditated on it and I took it very seriously, so periodically I attempt to win over my wife using my culinary arts. I have to admit that I have had some success, like my famous "mashed cauliflower" or my big "spicy guacamole." Before preparing my new culinary attempts I check a few cookbooks. In my collection there are three that stand out; one is entitled *1,000 Simple Recipes*, which has a misleading title, since they are not that simple. Then there are two others entitled *The Book of Creams* (which has some 150 recipes just for creams) and *The Big Book of Vegetarian Cooking*. My first step is to browse the recipe book and see what I like. Once I have selected the dish, I gather all the necessary ingredients that I will use, because if I want to make a cream of artichokes and I have no artichokes I would be in trouble.

DEFINITION OF A MENTAL DIAGRAM

A simple definition of a mental diagram would be:
"Visual structure with a central image in the middle from which the most important issues branch out."

What do artichokes have to do with mental diagrams? Well, I tried to create a simile. In this case we found a new recipe, that is to say, a new technique called mental diagrams. In the first chapter you were able to see what flavor it was, and if it looked appetizing you would have continued reading the book. But before we went into the kitchen to gather the ingredients, I enumerated them for you in the various chapters of this book. Our ingredients for creating mental diagrams are the right hemisphere, the left hemisphere, a handful of associations, and a high level of structuring. With these four ingredients we have enough to start cooking. But what is the recipe? Well, if you read on I will explain it step by step through a juicy example.

■ Step 1: **The central image**

In the definition of a mental diagram, there is an essential first element called the "central image." The term "central image" belongs to the specific nomenclature of mental diagrams and it refers to the first image we have to look for within us that relates to the issue that we will address.
To be able to see it, you must concentrate a bit, enter into alpha thinking, and try to visualize it. This is one of the most important points of creating mental diagrams. As with the visualization exercises, you have to start with the general shapes and then add all the additional details.

Do not try to have it be a logical and realistic picture; let your right hemisphere guide you. The richness of the image is very important because the more detail, the more associations you will make.

"The main idea is crystallized in the central image."

If you have a poor image you will get almost no associations. Try it out by doing a simple mental diagram of an orange. If the image is that of a circle, we will not find associations, or those we will find do not have much to do with an orange but rather with the circle. When the figure is too abstract the left hemisphere will take control and think something like "orange, juicy, and sweet." As you can see, there is too little information, and additionally, the left hemisphere may contradict itself and think something like "to be honest, an orange is not always sweet and juicy."

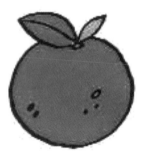

The picture of this orange tells us nothing; in fact, it could even be something else like a tomato or an apple.

What we have to look for is what an orange really means to us, and how we experience it. In this case here is an illustration depicting an orange for me. As I said, you have to unleash your imagination to the fullest, and this is what I clearly saw through the alpha thinking. Well, in my "vision" an orange greeted me, but I did not draw that, and I can also assure you that I did not take a psychotropic substance to visualize this juicy item.

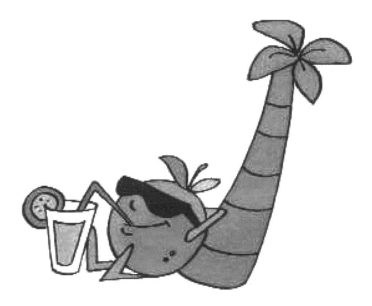

As you can see, this is the concept I visualized through alpha thinking. Isn't it amazing?

■ Step 2: Branched associations

Following along with the recipe, once we have the "vision" we have to re-create it in the center of a large landscape sheet. If you can, re-create the central image with colors and details, just as we talked about in the previous section. Now we will make a handful of associations. If you remember well, we already did several exercises where we sought associations, so this will not be a problem. Then add them freely around the central figure, and connect them with the so-called "branches." In the definition that I gave earlier in this chapter I spoke of "branched forms." This word is not random; the word "branch" is another of those mental diagrams keywords. Making a nice metaphor, we could say that the mind is like a tree diagram—the trunk is the central idea that connects through the branches with fruit, which in this case is the association. Is that not poetic?

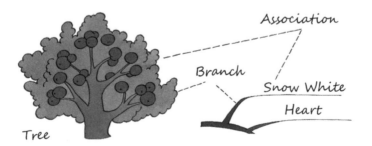

From the central image branches bear the fruit of associations.

For the example of an orange I had ten associations come to mind. As you can see, some were born out of the nature of the central image, because if we see the orange drinking an orange soda, that gives us some clues to the associations. You may think I watch too many cartoons, which is true, but the fact remains that using imagination gives life to the elements themselves, and that is what I have done with this orange.

Remember, as we saw in the chapter that mentioned the illustrious Sigmund Freud, we have to do an exercise of free association, without any censorship. At first I used this exercise with fruits while conducting mental diagrams workshops, so that each person could choose his or her favorite fruit. However, over time I saw that often bananas and melons were most often chosen. I am not a psychoanalyst, much less, but it is rather suspicious how often these fruits were chosen. Furthermore, when I asked for uncensored free associations, there were many with sexual content, so I changed the exercise and now I use an orange because I think it is more harmless.

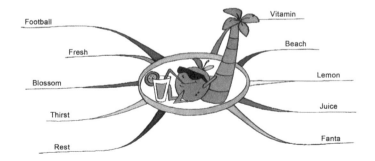

Mental diagram of an orange with the top ten most common associations

■ Step 3: **Ordered structures**

The third step to creating mental diagrams is to give it order. Its definition includes "important related issues." You will see that now there is a central figure and several associations, but they do not hold any special meaning. This is when we put to use what we learned about naturalistic intelligence. As the saying goes, "the trees keep you from seeing the forest," since we do not have a clear vision of the mental diagram. I hope you used a pencil to make this chart and you have an eraser handy, because you will need to use it. Now we will rearrange this information differently.

"It is important to use ranking and categorization to organize ideas."

Just as in the classification exercises, this is the time to organize branches in groups so that we can create categories. This is an essential step needed to simplify the mental diagrams. For example, we see that there are two words that have something in common: "juice" and "Fanta." Both are refreshing drinks, so we could create a category for them. Now we have to think about which word would be the best; maybe it is the word "soda" or the word "thirst," which already appeared in the first associations. In this case we will choose the word "thirst" and create that category. Within mental diagrams, this categorization has a special name; it is called the Basic Ordering Idea and it is usually referred to by its abbreviation BOI. This word that encompasses several elements must be selected with great care and precision. At this point you have to use your left hemisphere's full potential because having the right word will generate a powerful mental diagram. Now let us redo the diagram with the categories that we have found.

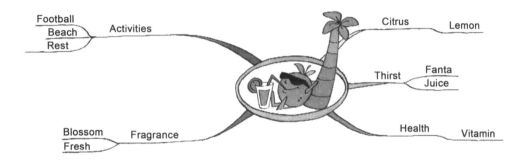

Mental diagram of an orange once the associations have been reorganized according to the basic ordering ideas

■ Step 4: **More associations and drawings**

Once you have organized the basic ordering ideas and their branches, you will sense a new creative flow, and when you see the categories you will start forming new associations. For example, in the associations that first appeared there was the word "lemon." That is perfectly fine because the lemon is closely related to an orange given that they are both drinks and citrus.

To be precise, we can create a basic ordering idea called "citrus." And in this new category we can add other citrus we know, like grapefruit, lime, tangerine, etc. It is also a good time to add more drawings and thus strengthen the mnemonic diagram.

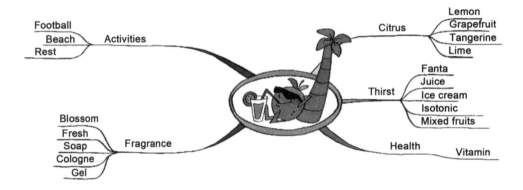

Through the basic ordering ideas found we can keep adding associations.

Well, what do you think? Amazing, right? As you can see, having all the ingredients makes the mental diagram recipe very simple; in fact, you already made some diagrams before almost without realizing it.

✌ ANSWERED QUESTIONS

Now that we have made our first complete mental diagram you will surely have questions. To save you the trouble of having to call me, I have compiled a small list of frequently asked questions that come up at this level.

✌ Why do you start with a large landscape sheet?

To begin the diagram we have to concentrate on the central image. This image has to be displayed graphically in the center of the sheet for the brain to realize its full potential freely in all directions, without restriction.

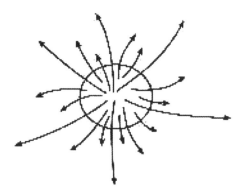

✌ Is it necessary to have a central image?

Yes, a picture is worth a thousand words. The image has hundreds of words that push the boundaries of your imagination. A central image is much more interesting than a word, and it will help you concentrate better.

✌ Should we use colors?

Yes, colors excite your imagination. By using colors you tickle the right hemisphere and wake it from its slumber. Colors add life and energy to a mental diagram. They are also very important because colors are much more amusing.

✌ Why is it necessary to connect the pictures and words through branches?

As you will remember, the brain works by making associations and these associations create links between ideas. On paper we re-create the deep structure of the brain and therefore we also express this union graphically. If we fail to draw connections it would be very difficult to understand a mental diagram.

✌ Should we always draw curved branches?

The answer is yes. I have personally done diagrams with straight lines and they become more complicated to read. What is the reason for this phenomenon? It turns out that our right hemisphere falls asleep when looking at too many straight lines. These lines produce a hypnotic effect, like a mandala. By adding curves you will mimic figures in nature that attract its attention, and it will help your right hemisphere find itself.

✌ Is it true that you have to use few words?

Yes, simple words offer great flexibility to mental diagrams. Simple words generate many associations, while compound words, or worse yet phrases, are dead ends for making associations.

✌ Other than the central image, should we use other pictures?

Definitely. Keep in mind that pictures can replace thousands of words. With only ten images in your mental diagram you will save about 10,000 words, which is saying a lot.

◉ MENTAL DIAGRAMS BASIC EXERCISES

We have already seen how a mental diagram is created to its full extent. How do you feel about making a couple of simple mental diagrams to warm up?

◉ Exercise number 1: USA

As you may very well remember, we did a similar exercise with Alaska. Back then, you did not know much about mental diagrams, but now you are an expert. Make a mental diagram of the United States, but based on my experience I can tell you that here you will have a lot of associations to choose from. I suggest that you:

1. Visualize the central idea clearly and in detail.
2. Add about twenty associations, although surely you might easily make over 200 (I speak from experience).
3. Rank and sort using the basic ordering ideas.

◉ Exercise number 2: The sea

A second exercise, which is also a lot of fun, is making a mental diagram of the sea. Obviously, in this case associations can also be infinite, so follow the same instructions as in the previous exercises but using the idea of "the sea."

GOALS OF THIS CHAPTER

The method

Mental diagrams require a series of steps to complete them. Each of these steps requires specific skills that we previously trained: visualization, drawing, associations, and order. A mental diagram is an organized visual structure and at its center is a central image from which associated ideas irradiate.

The objectives of this chapter are:

- Know which steps to take to create a mental diagram.
- Learn the specific words of mental diagrams: central idea, branch, and basic ordering idea.
- Develop complete mental diagrams.

9 Recommendations for creating mental diagrams

Creating a mental diagram requires following some guidelines. These guidelines are not strict rules you have to follow but rather they are ways to maximize its potential.

In this chapter we will review some tips on imagery, words, and inner state of mind.

- **Young warriors**

- **About images**

- **About words**

- **Three problems related to mental diagrams**

Young warriors

In ancient Japan there lived Bokuden, a great saber master. One day he received a visit from a colleague. To introduce his colleague to his three children as well as to show him the level that they attained by following his teachings, Bokuden prepared a little ruse: he placed a water jug at the edge of a sliding door so that it would fall on the head of anyone who entered the room.

Sitting with his friend facing the door, Bokuden called his eldest son. When the boy was right at the door, he stopped. He slightly pushed the door open and grabbed the jar before entering. He entered, closed the door behind him, placed the jug where it had sat along the edge of the door, and greeted the Masters.

"This is my oldest son," Bokuden said smiling. "He has already reached a good level and is poised to become a Master."

Then he called his second son. This boy slid the door open and started to enter. He dodged the jug that nearly fell on his skull, but managed to catch it in midair.

"This is my second child," he explained to the guest. "He still has a long way to go."

The third boy rushed in as he was called and the jug fell heavily on his neck, but before it hit the ground he drew his sword and broke it in two.

"And this," said the Master, "is my youngest son. He is the shame of the family, but he is still young."

Well, grasshopper, what is this little story's lesson? Initially, you will be in the place of the youngest child, eager to make mental diagrams but lacking the eldest son's great skill. How can you achieve this mastery? In two ways: the path of experience and the path of wisdom. The path of experience is a hard road in which you will have to make dozens of diagrams to begin discovering their tricks on your own. The path of wisdom is based on listening to the teacher's lesson (in this case the book) and skipping the experimentation that involves making dozens of diagrams to discover its secrets. Which is the best path? As wise teachers say: neither or both. The answer lies in the middle path; practice without knowledge is slow, but knowledge without practice is sterile. What am I suggesting in this chapter? Learn a few tricks that will help you become the master of mental diagrams.

About images

The picture

As we have seen, images are a key element in the creation of mental diagrams. You have to rid your mind of the fear of drawing. Although I explain the importance of the drawings, I have often seen with great sadness that new mental cartographers tend to use very little artwork, and this is a serious mistake. By not using drawings to create mental diagrams you miss their magic and you end up with very simple diagrams. If at first your pictures do not turn out as well as you expected, do not get impatient. Drawing is a matter of practice, and at first it is difficult to see objects with new eyes. Keep in mind that drawing is like reopening your eyes to the world.

Color

A second issue related to the drawings is color. I have met people who use drawings in their mental diagrams, but they have a hard time giving them color. I understand that there are people with vision problems and they have difficulty distinguishing colors (as it happens to me), but I do not think that this happens to most people. Almost all human beings are ready to perceive the richness of color. Would you rather see the world in black and white or in color? In light of the low interest in black and white TVs, and the high popularity of color televisions, I am inclined to think that you would prefer colors in the world and also in your mental diagrams. Color represents life, emotion, and energy, so it would be unfair to deprive them of all that. Imagine a monochrome diagram, with a single color, dull, monotonous—it would be terrible! Remember to add a little color to your life.

Dimension

A third issue related to the drawings is dimension. I have also frequently observed that when someone who is learning mental diagrams succeeds in making his first drawings, he forgets the dimension. Encouraged by the clear

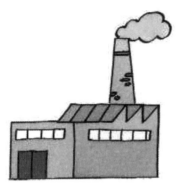
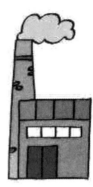

Which of these two factories do you think is more interesting to the eye, the two-dimensional or the three-dimensional?

schematic representations he makes, he is convinced that he has reached the limits of his artistic ability. Nothing is further from the truth—once you get the right shape you must give it volume. This is the master level in our quick drawing course. Usually, the objects we see are three-dimensional, so why not represent the images in our mental diagrams the same way?

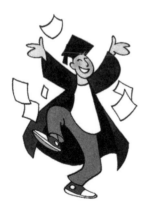

An emphasized representation of the moment in which I ended my college career

Self-expression

A fourth and final issue related to drawing is self-expression. If we make realistic drawings, we may not quite convey the emotion we want to capture, so a useful trick is to emphasize the drawing. For instance, to represent a sad person, we would draw someone who is very sad, perhaps crying or kneeling on the floor, or even asking for help. Conversely, if we want to express joy or excitement we will have to draw this person in a way that leaves no room for doubt about his emotions. Do not be afraid to exaggerate the expressiveness of the drawing.

"Drawing pictures with strong and expressive colors is essential for creating mental diagrams."

About words

As we saw in the previous chapter, the correct word choice is necessary. If we choose it well, we will be able to maximize the associations. Otherwise we will close ourselves off to many options.

Legibility

The first problem that I have observed in the creation of mental diagrams is the illegibility of our letters. I myself have found some of my old mental diagrams with incomprehensible writing, and I wasted time and concentration trying to figure out what the hell I meant. I recommend that you always try to write clearly, and if it is possible you should print. This matters because we need

Excerpt from the manuscript of one of my books. Would you be able to decipher what it says?

to be able to understand what we put down, but also because we should avoid having to decipher our intentions. Some people have come to me arguing that if they make their words more legible they will work at a slower pace and thus lose their creative flow. But if you write illegibly you will also lose time and focus, so I leave it up to you to decide how you want to approach it.

Size

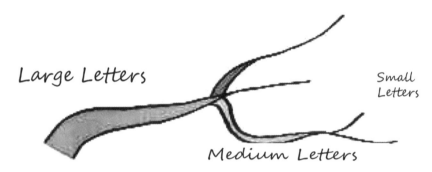

The sizes of the letters and branches must match.

A second factor that hinders the power of mental diagrams is the font size. As the new mental cartographer gets into it, he could be making a mistake: writing all the words the same size. The idea of mental diagrams is to make the main branches (those with the basic ordering ideas) thicker than the secondary branches. This choice is not random because it regards the readability criteria. If you look at a well-built mental diagram you should be able to understand its main points at a glance. How is that possible? Because the thickness of the main branches indicates the most important ideas, and those important ideas are written in big letters.

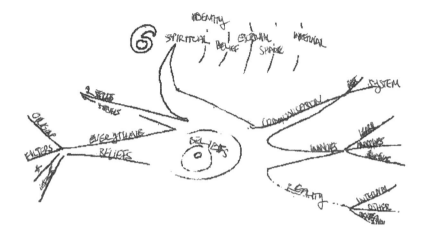

Can you tell what is right and what is wrong with this mental diagram?

Three problems related to mental diagrams

I have personally taught countless mental diagrams workshops and I always ask myself the same question: If the attendees understand the ideas and find this technique interesting, why do they not apply it more often? After asking countless questions and giving serious thought to this issue, I have come to the following conclusion: the main enemies of mental diagrams are anxiety, lack of concentration, and lack of confidence in them. Often these problems do not happen separately; they appear together, or they are brought on by one another. For example, some people want to make an excellent mental diagram, but the notion that they might not be able to achieve it makes them feel a lot of anxiety and that fear paralyzes them. Sometimes lack of concentration keeps them from getting the expected results so they give up learning the technique. For other cartographers, the lack of confidence in themselves or a lack of confidence in the technique makes them give up this technique altogether. They conclude that in one way or another this technique is impaired, so that its usefulness is minimal. What can we do about these problems?

"Three major difficulties you may encounter: anxiety, lack of concentration, and lack of confidence."

---

1. Anxiety

To overcome anxiety we will practice using the right hemisphere. Typically, anxiety manifests itself through various internal messages that we constantly give ourselves, telling us that we will not achieve our desired results. The solution is to transform these negative messages into much more positive ones. To this end we can practice the exercise in chapter 2 called "The Senate" and try to find out who gives us these messages and why. Another thing to try is to go into alpha thinking to dissolve this messenger along with its words. In this state we can visualize ourselves making the mental diagram with a positive, enthusiastic, and cheerful attitude.

2. Concentration

We currently bear many responsibilities on our shoulders. Our lives are complex and we have to respond to countless commitments. What happens to all this pressure? Our mind becomes a hive of chaotic ideas that are out of control. With a scattered mind, any attempt to create a mental diagram is an almost impossible mission. What can we do? We can apply the skills learned to managing our thoughts and focusing on a task. A key to good concentration is displaying our diagram's central image. Before starting a mental diagram we must dedicate enough time to reviewing the central image for our project. If you visualize this image the right way, your entire brain and your attention will work toward creating the mental diagram and your ideas will be able to sprout naturally. If you do not achieve this level of concentration, repeat the relaxation practices described in chapters 2 and 3.

3. Confidence

Trust is hard to get and easy to lose. How do we become confident? Mainly through two ways: by faith and by experience. I am not asking you to blindly believe in mental diagrams, although that would be helpful, but do consider the practices that we have done. If you have practiced them all you will have noticed little by little the power hidden in the mind and the solutions that the mental diagrams offer. In fact, by now you must have made at least four or five mental diagrams.

INTERNAL AND EXTERNAL DISTRACTION

One thing that destabilizes us in the task of making a mental diagram is the issue of distraction. There could be two types of distraction: internal and external. Internal distraction respond to what we experience in our inner state, such as thoughts about weekend plans. External distraction are much easier to control than the former. They are as simple as trying to do a mental diagram in front of the television or during a party. I will not elaborate much on this but I will give you several tips that will help you streamline your energy toward the interesting task of creating mental diagrams.

- Prepare all the materials you will need.
- Take advantage of daylight whenever possible.
- Do not make mental diagrams while watching TV or listening to music that can distract you.
- Plan how much time you will spend making the mental diagram.
- Find a comfortable and relaxed place to work at ease.
- Do not fall asleep while visualizing.
- Be sure that the room you are in has adequate ventilation so that oxygen can get to the brain.
- Sit in a comfortable chair that supports your back and maintain proper posture.

After everything you have seen, do you think they can be useful to you? Do you think they can benefit your work development? You must have answered these questions affirmatively. Think about your own experience and you will see that working with mental diagrams is worth doing.

GOALS OF THIS CHAPTER

Recommendations

Mental diagrams hide some dangers. Some are related to images, since there is a tendency to use a few colorless drawings with little emotion. On the other hand, when words are used there is a tendency to write illegible, same-size, and crooked letters. Lastly, your internal state is very important when making a mental diagram. You need to be focused, attentive, and relaxed at the same time.

The objectives of this chapter are:

- Remember the importance of using expressive images.
- Include words of different sizes that correspond to different hierarchical levels in the diagram.
- Develop the right mental attitude to successfully create a mental diagram.

Applications

Now that we know how to create and structure mental diagrams we will put them to use. In this third section there are three general areas where the mental diagrams technique has been applied successfully:

The first area is the personal level, with a strong analytical component. In this section we will see how to create an agenda, how to make decisions, and how to conduct self-analysis, all via mental diagrams (Ch. 10).

The second analyzed area revolves around teaching. In this area the memory skills that we acquire are very important. Mental diagrams will teach us their extensive organizational and mnemonic potential through book summaries and note-taking (Ch. 11).

The third evaluated area is at the business level. Mental diagrams will demonstrate their creative potential through projects, reports, and conferences (Ch. 12).

10 Personal decisions

Can mental diagrams help us with personal matters? In what ways can we use them? In this section, we will explore personal life decisions and offer three applications: an agenda, a decision-making method, and self-analysis.

■ **My brain cannot handle any more**

■ **A rational being**

■ **An agenda, decision making, and self-analysis**

■ My brain cannot handle any more

Undoubtedly, thinking is hard work and an expensive activity that many like to avoid. Of course there are all types of thoughts; it is very different to think about what you want for breakfast than to think about what you want to do with your life. However, both require some degree of effort and determination. If you pay attention to a normal day in your life you will see that you are constantly faced with choices. As soon as the alarm clock goes off, you have to decide what to eat for breakfast, what to wear, and most importantly, if you are actually going to go to work or if you are going to call in sick. Well, as you can see, you have not even left your house and have already had to make several decisions. And whether you decide to stay at home or go to work, you will still have to make dozens of decisions that day. No wonder people are exhausted with so much mental effort and they do not want to keep thinking, which is something that happens more often than we would like. Do we really think about what we do?

■ A rational being

If you were a perfect and rational being, you would have no problem making decisions. You would rate the information coldly and you would choose the most practical and effective option, just as a robot or a computer would. However, we are not cold but warm-blooded, and sometimes we make decisions with our heart or stomach. What is certain is that our decisions are influenced by our feelings.

DO YOU WANT LIFE INSURANCE?

One technique that is often explained in books and lectures is the listing technique. According to this technique, you have to make a list of a decision's pros and cons. The lists are compared and the one with more elements wins. This would be a rational decision-making model. However, it is one of the least rational methods. Many salesmen use this technique for their potential clients to decide. The trick is that the order in which the list begins is very important, because the first list always has many more elements than the second one. Thus, the salesman starts with the "pros of buying life insurance," and as you can imagine, there are hardly any cons.

Oftentimes, in our decision-making process there are elements that are not rational: mysterious elements such as hunches, intuitions, or worse yet, the hunches and intuitions of others. The left hemisphere would be happy to make every decision using its overwhelming logic, but its twin hemisphere interferes. If your corpus callosum was sectioned there would be no problem, but the likelihood that you have undergone surgery is low. Apparently, our right hemisphere has opinions and even makes decisions without the use of words.

■ An agenda, decision making, and self-analysis

Would it be possible to make decisions by integrating as much information as possible and taking into account both rational and emotional factors? The answer is a clear and resounding yes. And best of all, you now know the technique to achieve this. If you look closely, the mental diagrams method fits perfectly in the complicated decision-making process:

1. Integrates the right hemisphere and the left hemisphere
2. Processes and values a wealth of information
3. Creates order and hierarchy among the data

If we had all the elements that are involved in decision making organized in a clear and orderly manner, it would be very easy to choose the right path.

In this chapter entitled "Personal decisions" we will use the mental diagrams technique for three types of personal applications:

→   AN AGENDA
    (How do I organize and decide the things that need to get done?)

→   DECISION MAKING IN PERSONAL MATTERS
    (Do I have to buy a new car?)

→   SELF-ANALYSIS
    (What do I want to do with my life?)

By looking at these three applications, you will see that they have something in common; the three applications share two characteristics, the common denominator of this section:

1. A heavy situation analysis.
2. Making a decision that will determine our course of action for a day, a few years, or our entire lives.

→ THE AGENDA

The first point of introduction into the practical applications of mental diagrams is the agenda. I do not know if you ever used the typical planner given at the beginning of each year. I have collected several of them and I only ever manage to fill in January. From there, the agenda stays buried in books until it expires and it joins its companions from previous years.

The mental diagrams theory suggests making an agenda in the style of a mental diagram. Using it will allow you to decide what you want to do with all the information. The problem with the old agendas was that the left hemisphere dominated them. In them were words, numbers, lists, and order, but they forgot about pictures, color, dreams, associations, and visualization.

Using an agenda in the style of a mental diagram is the same as creating a standard mental diagram, just like the one we created using the orange. Do you want to see an example? Well, let us see what I have to do this week.

This week I have to . . .

For work, I sometimes have to travel to other cities to lecture and teach courses, and this will be one of those weeks. It is also time to pay taxes, which is something that complicates my schedule. I also have to buy a tire for my son's bike, because it is flat and he has been calling me about it every day for more than a month. Anyway, as you can see I have many commitments this week, but first things first.

CENTRAL IMAGE

In the central image I see myself on the flight that I have to take on July 29. As this is a key date in the week, I am using it as a point of reference, and the vision that I have of the plane is something like this. My papers are flying away. Traveling on one of its wings is not very comfortable, but it is cheap.

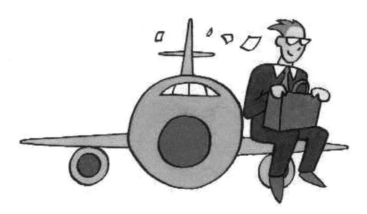

BRAINSTORM

According to the method we studied, we now have to brainstorm quickly, write down whatever comes to mind, without any order, randomly and rapidly. You will see all sorts of topics appear, some as minimal as having to buy toothpaste and others that are more important such as purchasing airline tickets. From the central figure itself there is one of the most important elements of the week, the trip (tickets, hotel, preparing for the conference, etc.). Well, for now I have jotted down twenty-three commitments.

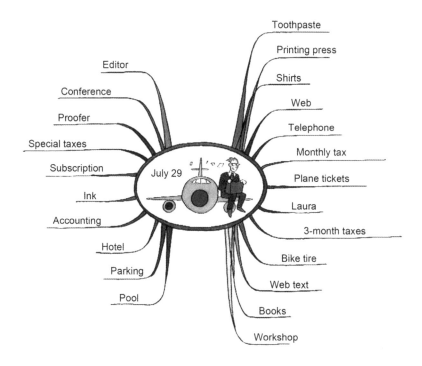

REORGANIZATION

Now because this diagram is so chaotic we will start to put it in order. As always, we begin to form groups according to similarity: a group that comes out right away is a shopping section. Another important group is travel related, particularly because without tickets or hotel reservations I will not get very far. Similarly the rest of the commitments continue gathering until they have an acceptable order. Perhaps this illustration does not look very good, but it is color-coded: I assigned the lighter colors to more pleasant tasks such as leisure, sorting, and studying (at least for me). The serious topics have black branches, and in this case they are for the trip and paying all taxes. The rest (purchases, meeting, contact, and work) is colored in red.

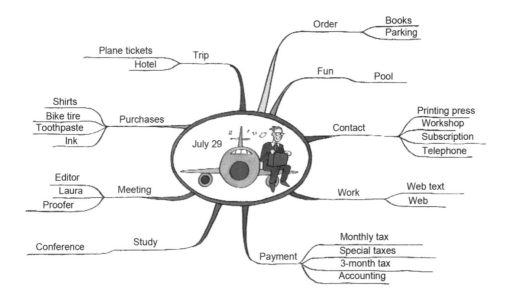

What do you think? In less than five minutes I organized a series of important things that worried me, and now in the mental diagram they are clear and organized. Now all I have to do is determine on which days I will do each task, revise it, and cross off what I get done; isn't that great?

👁 **Exercise number 1: The week's agenda**

As you may have guessed, there is an interesting exercise waiting for you. It is called the week's agenda and it is as simple as making your own agenda. You have seen how I made mine, so go ahead; you will see how useful this is.

Other Uses

As I already explained, you can apply the agenda in the style of a mental diagram for other related uses, such as:

- Planning family events.
- Organizing a romantic weekend.
- Making a shopping list (very useful indeed).

WHAT CAN AN AGENDA IN THE STYLE OF A MENTAL DIAGRAM PROVIDE US?

- A wide and at the same time narrow vision of life that gives us the flexibility to organize.
- A visually appealing way to plan commitments.
- A powerful mnemonic device.

→ DECISION MAKING

Mental diagrams have many advantages for analyzing decisions such as making a purchase or changing jobs. Mental diagrams take into account both the rational (priorities and constraints) as well as the emotional elements (needs and desires).

The mental diagram process

Suppose you are planning to buy a new car. For this, we start to visualize the central image about the possibility of buying a new car. Since this is about evaluating a decision, we will take two basic ordering ideas to begin our diagram: yes and no.

If we had a good visualization, we will have a picture full of life that will guide us toward making multiple associations to the pros and cons. At this point, you have to let the thoughts about the possible purchase flow freely. Once you have run out of associations, you have to sort the ideas for and against according to their level of importance. Once you rearrange them you will see that it is possible that the "tree" is asymmetrical and that one of its major branches (yes or no) shifted the balance. In such a case, the decision will have been made.

Two items to note: a little storm and a lot of emotions

There are two elements related to this type of diagram that are worth
mentioning. The first is that it is not necessary to maximize the branches
of the basic ordering ideas. This means that we do not have to expand the
diagram to its limits. The reason for this is that the most important elements,
both for and against, came out during the first brainstorm. If you then force
yourself to make more factors appear, I doubt that they will come out, but if
they do then their relevance is low or minimal. If we carelessly include them,
we may end up creating a falsely unbalanced tree.

The second element related to decision-making mental diagrams has to do
with color. Throughout the book we placed great emphasis on the issue of
colors, and now this element is important, but for another reason, for its
ability to convey emotions. It is very important to utilize colors because
the emotions you have associated with the different factors are expressed
through them. By using them, you will easily see what kind of emotions are
involved in your decision-making process.

Do I have to buy a motorcycle?

A few months ago, I contemplated the idea of buying a motorcycle. Until now,
I have been driving my car to work. I live far from the city, in the countryside,
and to commute I need a comfortable vehicle with good mileage. For my
leisure, I have an old rusty bicycle that still has a couple of years left.

However, I have always wanted to have a motorcycle to ride in my spare time. The bike is not the same because I cannot get very far riding it, and despite having an athletic body (I am 5'9" and weigh 143 pounds) I do not like pedaling around. How could I decide if I should buy a motorcycle?

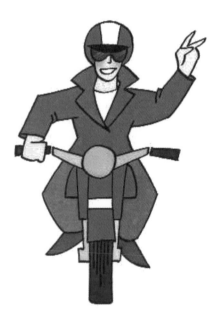

THE CENTRAL IMAGE

We will start by focusing and visualizing the central idea. In this case I see myself on the motorcycle, all happy and satisfied. Also, the motorcycle that I want does not have large cylinders, it is just to roam the countryside, and that is the idea that I wanted to transmit in this drawing.

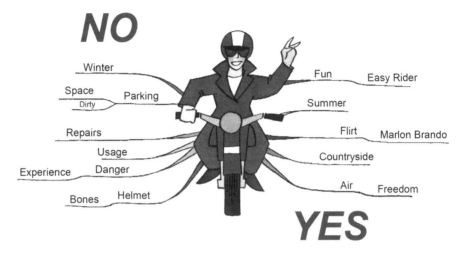

Mental diagram brainstorming

BRAINSTORM

Now that I have a central image, it is time to seek associations. I have the first ones ready because they are included in the drawing itself. I look pretty happy on the motorcycle. I think of fun and the wind on my face. I also think of summer and everything seems idyllic. And through associations, I could also see myself flirting more if I owned a motorcycle because I never meet girls while riding my bicycle. The only one who dared to join me for a ride (after much pleading) was my wife who after ten yards of riding with me jumped off the bike and said she would never do that again. But I have to be honest and acknowledge the cons (if there were none, I would have already bought it). I've never owned a motorcycle before and I know nothing about its maintenance. Also, I will not be able to use it year-round, as the winter here is very cold and it would be reckless to drive around in those temperatures.

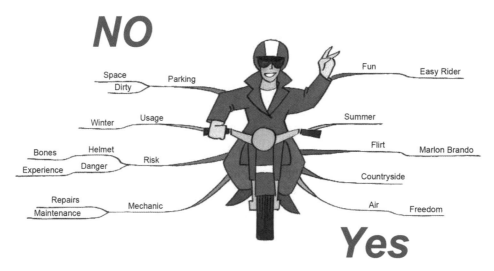

Reorganized mental diagram

I do not have a place to park a motorcycle, and as I keep thinking about it, I see that there is a great probability of getting into an accident. Well, this is just a brainstorm; the most important thing is to write all the pros and cons, while being realistic and honest at the same time.

REORGANIZATION

Now that we have all the associations ready we need to organize the mental diagram according to the BOI. Once the classification is done you can see that in the diagram the factors against are more organized and seem more powerful than those in favor. Even so, it still lacks something from the point of view of the right hemisphere—colors and an emotional charge. Will there be any changes?

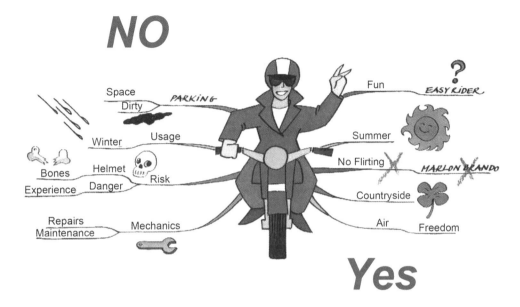

Mental diagram with emotional elements included

BRINGING IT TO LIFE

Now that everything is more organized, I will try to add colors and pictures to assess what "my heart" is really telling me. Well, more than my heart, I have to listen to my right hemisphere. In reviewing the good points I see no clear images. On the first item I see "Easy Rider" appear, and there is the image of the film's protagonist on the motorcycle, but I do not see myself traveling great distances and having all kinds of adventures; rather I see this as an unknown. Another striking point is the topic of flirting. If I were to show my wife this diagram I doubt she would like it, and if she were to see me on the motorcycle with a girl, she would like it even less. And since I want to continue having a good relationship with her (at least for the time being), I better get rid of this branch. The few pros that remain are minimal because I already get fresh air (riding the bicycle), I live in the countryside and summer will be over quickly, or I might have to stay indoors working.

But if we look at the cons, the images are much clearer. I see a crowded parking space with a dirty floor covered in oil stains. I also see the motorcycle parked and left unused all winter long. I also see broken bones, or something worse. I also see myself trying to learn its maintenance and getting frustrated.

Well, in short, you do not need to be a genius to realize that at least this year I will not get a motorcycle. It is true that I will always have the bicycle, although it is starting to hurt my knees because it is not the right size for me. In fact, if I could raise the saddle, it would be a lot more comfortable.

Thus, my decision is made, or at least postponed for another time when the pros are in fact much more clear and more powerful than the cons.

◎ **Exercise number 2: A decision has to be made**
As you can see, making decisions with the use of mental diagrams is fairly quick and practical. And now it is your turn: start by thinking of something that you have been wanting to buy for some time but you still have not, for one reason or another. Create a decision-making mental diagram and find out which opinions and emotions hide behind your indecision.

Other selection modes

The faster selection mode is based on having the diagram itself work as a balance that will have most of its weight on either side. However, there are other types of selections that can be made using the mental diagram. Such possibilities are:

1. Spontaneous generation: It is possible that while we are concocting a mental diagram we get inspired, and suddenly the decision we need becomes very clear. Some people say this is like some sort of enlightenment or revelation.

2. Numerical rating: This will be especially appealing to people who have clear rationalistic tendencies. This method consists in scoring the BOI with points for the pros and points against the cons. Each positive branch will have a score between 1 and 100. On the other hand, the negative branches will score between -1 and -100. Then you add both sides and whichever has the highest score wins.

3. Enhanced intuition: Sometimes after creating and evaluating the diagram, you may still disagree with it. This is not because you did the process incorrectly but rather because there are factors that are difficult to express. The right hemisphere is certainly trying to tell us something, but it has no specific words or convincing arguments. Still, you have to give it a chance.

HOW CAN MENTAL DIAGRAMS HELP US MAKE DECISIONS?

- They allow us to absorb large amounts of related complex information so that we can focus more clearly on the conflicting issues.
- They bring colors and images that project our emotions associated with each different option.
- The analytical process itself triggers a decision.
- It generates a wider range of related elements than any other type of technique.

4. With a stroll: Many times, making a decision is a totally exhausting process. Having to decide any important issue is often synonymous with getting overwhelmed by the effort because, after all, many decisions determine our future. So if you feel fatigued by the effort, the best thing you can do is relax and take a stroll. This will help ease the tension you are feeling because of your concentration on the problem, and you will give yourself some time for the right hemisphere to help you understand the problem without thinking about it in-depth. Try it and you will see how useful it is.

→ SELF-ANALYSIS

As I explained in chapter 1, there are mental diagrams that can help you discover who you are. These mental diagrams are for self-analysis. They are designed to get a better understanding of yourself and your environment: you will be able to easily visualize who you are and who you want to be.

Steps for making a mental diagram for self-analysis
1. PREPARATION

Before starting your own mental diagram, you must carefully consider where you are going to do this task. Keep in mind the advice that I gave you when we discussed external and internal distractions. When it comes to something as important as self-analysis, your environment should be comfortable and enjoyable.

2. CENTRAL IMAGE

Relax, go into alpha state, and visualize yourself. Let your mind make an extensive tour of your different daily activities, your past, and the things that matter to you. Also think about how you are, what characterizes you, in short, anything that can help you visualize a central image. Once you have it, draw it in the center of the sheet and remember to add life and color to it.

3. BRAINSTORM

Now that you have a picture that represents who you are, you must do some free association. It is important to work very fast here, even if it does not turn out too neatly. Find associations and let experiences, ideas, and emotions appear on their own. Remember that it is also very useful to include personality traits and add them to the diagram. Sometimes there are personal conflicts. It is good to let them emerge and evaluate them in the diagram because they are a part of you and representing them will bring you closer to the solution.

4. RECONSTRUCTION

After brainstorming there is a time for reconstruction. We have to find the basic ordering ideas to group our branches.

By the very nature of the mental diagram, a few key categories will often appear. I have listed them for you so that they can help you select a few BOIs for your groupings:

Personal history	Strengths
Weaknesses	Achievements
What you like	What you dislike
Hobbies	Emotions
Family	Friends
Problems	Long-term objectives
Health	Work

5. REFLECTION

Looking at the finished mental diagram, you can already analyze "who you are" and make the right decisions that will steer you toward "who you want to be."

Exercise number 3: Who am I?

In this exercise we will create a mental diagram for self-analysis. There is no reason for you to be afraid because they tend to be more entertaining and enjoyable than other diagrams. Do it according to the instructions described in this section and I am sure that besides getting a pleasant surprise, you will be able to clarify many ideas about yourself.

WHAT CAN SELF-ANALYSIS DIAGRAMS PROVIDE US?

- Develop a more objective vision of ourselves.
- Provide a comprehensive and detailed view of the person.
- Facilitate future planning.
- Having designs and colors facilitates emotional expression.

---

11 Teaching

Memory is an important element for training and education. There are many methods for remembering information, but there is one that stands out among the rest—it is mental diagrams. In this section we will study the mnemonic functions of mental diagrams and see two practical applications: books summaries and note-taking.

■ **I forgot**

■ **The nodal model**

■ **Mnemonics**

■ **Summarizing a book and note-taking**

■ I forgot

Have you ever forgotten a phone number you just dialed? Has your mind ever gone blank while taking a test? Did you greet someone you met but you cannot remember his or her name?

These situations are all imperfections in our memory, our unpredictable system of information storage and retrieval. But while it is often imperfect, it is also true that sometimes it has amazing features. Often it retains accurate memories of things that happened weeks, years, or even decades ago!

■ The nodal model

One of the classic models for understanding memory is the nodal model. According to this model, we have not a single memory but three different memory systems. The first is sensory memory, which temporarily stores the information provided by our senses. The second type is the short-term memory, which retains relatively small amounts of information for a short period of time (usually 30 seconds or less). This is the memory we use when we see a phone number and dial it right away. The third type is our long-term memory, which allows us to retain large amounts of information for long periods of time.

This model answers an interesting question: How do we transfer information from one system to another? Apparently, we have a series of filters that allow information to go from one memory bank into another. There are some "active control processes" that act as filters determining what information is retained. Information enters the sensory memory through the short-term memory when it becomes a focus of our attention; sensory impressions that do not get our focused attention vanish and disappear quickly. Thus, the process of paying attention is key for sensory information to go into the short-term memory. And how does it go from the short-term to the long-term memory? The transfer occurs when there is an "elaborative review." When we think of short-term information seeking meaning in it and relating it to other information we already have stored in our long-term memory is when the transfer occurs.

Selective attention: It is the ability to pay attention only to some aspects of the world around us, ignoring the rest.

■ Mnemonics

While the nodal theory explains how different memory banks are connected through attention and significance, it does not explain how we can better remember. Along with these theories, ways in which we can better remember phone numbers, addresses, or even complicated formulas have always been sought. From this search comes mnemonics, which is "the art of increasing memory retention."

Mnemonics mainly provide techniques to memorize and recall lists of names, numbers, strings, speeches, etc. A common method used in all these types of techniques is relying on the imagination, association, and visualization. Using these tools new images are created and easily remembered. But if we pay attention to these tools, it is clear that they are almost the same used in the creation of mental diagrams. In mental diagrams we find the two hemispheres working together through images, associations, words, and structures. Therefore, mnemonic mental diagrams are identical, both in mechanism and design, to the mental diagrams we already know. Can mental diagrams dramatically increase our memory retention? The answer is affirmative.

■ Summarizing a book and note-taking

Within this chapter about teaching we will apply the mnemonic mental diagrams technique to:

→   SUMMARIZE A BOOK
→   TAKE NOTES

What do these applications have in common? Well, both contain a large volume of information that should be well structured, but the most outstanding feature is that both should be easily stored in the long-term memory. Although all mental diagrams have a great mnemonic load, we are particularly interested in using it to its fullest capacity.

→ BOOK SUMMARY

You have probably read several books with ideas you found interesting. They may have been technical books, developmental, or any other topic. In all these books you found a handful of theories, practices, and ideas that you wish you could remember, but memory is whimsical and it is unlikely that they moved from your short-term to your long-term memory. Well, that is not a problem; here we will suggest a method of summarizing a book using a mental diagram: amazing but true.

Phases for summarizing a book

The book summary is divided into three phases. The first phase is called preparation. Here we will concentrate on skimming the book, finding the main image, and using our knowledge on the subject. The second phase is actually reading and completely designing the mental diagram. And the third phase is reviewing the mental diagram to store it in the long-term memory.

Preparation phase

1. INITIAL GLANCE

Before you start reading the book you have to get a feel for it. To do this you need to get an overview of it, flip through the index, look at its cover, read the back, see if it has illustrations and diagrams, read the biography of the author (if any), etc. At this stage the most important thing is to get a general feel of the book.

After this thorough review you have to search for the central image, focus, and visualize it. If the book cover has an image that is meaningful, you should use it.

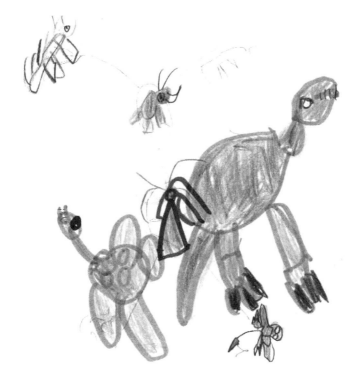

Mental diagram about dinosaurs made by a four-year-old. The central image is an erupting volcano.

If you also know what the main branches (BOI) of the book will be, this is a good time to add them to the diagram. They often correspond to the major segments of the book, which usually appear in the table of contents.

2. EXISTING KNOWLEDGE

At this stage we have to dump information onto a quick mental diagram. Grab a new sheet and make a mental diagram with all that you know about the topic. Do it as fast as your pencil will allow. You may end up with what was captured in the book that you want to summarize as well as other similar or related sources. The purpose of this exercise is to bring out all the information you already have and to start the process of association with the subject. Additionally, it will help you identify the strengths and weaknesses of your knowledge of this subject.

3. OBJECTIVES

It may be interesting to add to this diagram some branches that address the reasons that made you want to summarize this book and the objectives you hope to achieve. Mapping the objectives makes the brain more sensitive to the information related to your interests.

Application phase

Now we have two mental diagrams—first there is a draft on which you put the associations and knowledge you already possess, and then a second diagram that still needs to be completed with words, pictures, and concepts. Then we have to read and map—it is that simple.

4. PREVIEW

In the preview, browse whatever you think you can read in one sitting. Make an estimate of the time available and how much you can cover in that amount of time. Whenever possible, you should finish a significant information block in that sitting. Now that you looked over the chosen block (photos, titles, diagrams) you are ready to start reading.

5. READING

Look for a quiet place and try to be focused enough to understand what you are reading. Limit your time and try to enjoy the text. If you think you have concentration problems use the exercises outlined in chapter 2.

6. MAPPING

Now you can map out what you have read. Think of the chapters, what has grabbed your attention, and the associations you found. It is important that your diagram include opinions and impressions that you had while reading the text. Recording these ideas will help you make mnemonic associations.

Review phase

When you start reviewing the mental diagram a lot of elements that are present in your long-term memory may start to appear. You should also perform an "elaborative review" to store information in the long-term memory. Think of it as a game, check the mental diagram carefully examining the drawings and colors, and ask yourself the meaning of the different branches. Then with all your visualization powers, close your eyes and hold it in your memory. Observe its general shape and then go over the various items that comprise it, its drawings, its words, and its associations. You will see that the mental diagram will remain in a database for a long time.

An example: theories about memory

There was a time when I studied the memory of a great university book simply called *Psychology*. Throughout its 800 pages, the book unfolds the mysteries of the psyche. Even today I look at it with curiosity and satisfaction because it is very well written and entertaining. Part of the cognitive processes are explained in chapter 6, entitled "Memory: of things remembered . . . and forgotten." I have long wanted to make a mental diagram of the chapter, and I finally had the chance.

FIRST LOOK

Before starting the diagram, I looked over the chapter and I got a good idea of it. After browsing the topic, I thought about the mental image. In this case it was a bit difficult since there were many. One I had in mind was a brain inside a glass jar, but when I drew it I did not really like it. Then I thought of a guy who looked at his own brain with wonder, and even though that may sound a bit icky I thought it looked good, and that was the one I chose. Thereupon I made the sections I wanted (BOI); in this case there were two models (parallel processing and the linear model), memory type classification and a section on "the act of remembering."

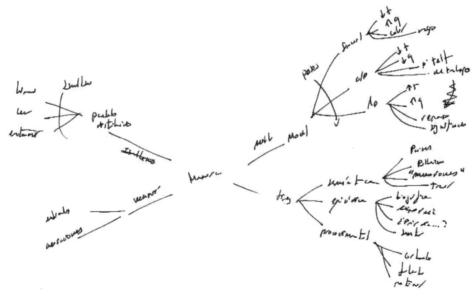

Rough draft of existing knowledge

EXISTING KNOWLEDGE

I also made a brief diagram of the knowledge I had about the subject, and there were many, albeit a bit confusing.

OBJECTIVES

Actually, there were many interesting topics, but unfortunately not all were within my goal, which was just to pick out a couple of good models and a memory typology.

For this reason, from the beginning I discarded the segment about memory disorders (amnesia, Korsakoff's syndrome, or Alzheimer's disease, for example).

There were also some other things that did not interest me, and others that were too intricate.

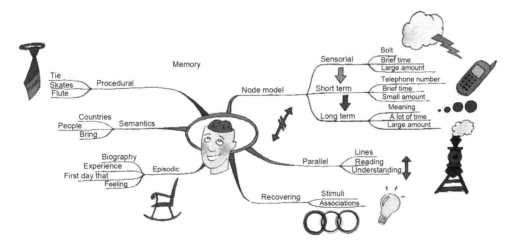

Complete diagram on the topic of memory

PREVIEW AND READING

While reading the book I wrote down ideas and words that came to me until I finished the chapter.

MAPPING

Once I had the basic information, I redid the mental diagram just as it is shown in the illustration. In it I could find some examples that appear in the book, such as the tie to explain procedural memory; others I made up, such as the parallel memory model, which is represented by the train tracks (according to this model, information is processed at the same time but at different levels).
If you look at it closely enough, you will see that it covers the objectives I set: the two models I want to study, the classification, and a section about retrieving memories.

HOW CAN MENTAL DIAGRAMS HELP ME TO SUMMARIZE BOOKS?

- Have an overall picture of the knowledge that you have about the topic.
- They take up less space than linear summaries.
- Provide a clear structure to organizing knowledge.
- Relate the book's content to your own knowledge, ideas, and opinions.
- They are a powerful mnemonic tool due to their structure and associated imagery.
- Reinforce memory and understanding in a powerful, simple, and fun way.

👁 **Exercise number 1: A good book**

Find a book that has impacted you. It can be about alternative medicines, information processes, "Wicca," or even cooking. Leaf through it and see if there is a special chapter about which you want a mental diagram. Once you have it, all you have to do is create your mental diagram about the chapter in question. Follow the steps carefully and you will see that the result is a success.

→ NOTE TAKING

Surely you have been to events where it would have been helpful to take notes. If you are a student, taking notes is your job, but you might also have to take notes during work meetings or conferences.

Note taking is capturing someone else's ideas from an oral discourse and organizing them so that they reflect the author's thought. As we saw in chapter 1, it is the students' workhorse since they are used to taking notes in a monochromatic and linear manner. Taking notes should be a more personal task where associations, colors, opinions, and thoughts appear. Therefore, it shares some similarity to summarizing books as explained above.

The analytical function
Taking notes in a mental diagram requires identifying the information's underlying structure. Usually, when dealing with a book, the author has made a major formal text structuring so that it is clearly organized. The book is arranged into chapters, and each chapter has a specific objective.

But at conferences and lectures there may not be such a defined degree of structuring, so the challenge is to find it.

"The main function of taking notes is to identify the underlying structure of the speaker."

How to take notes
Just as in book summaries, taking notes has two phases: preparation and application. As we will see, the preparation phase is similar; however, there are marked differences in the application.

Preparation phase
The preparation phase is similar to that explained in the previous section. However, in this case you may not have a chance to browse the material before the lecture or the conference, so we will focus on the information load and on defining the objectives. The procedure for developing them is explained in the section on book summaries.

- Setting up existing knowledge
- Annotation of objectives

Application phase
This second phase is quite different from the section on book summaries, but it follows the same principles. At this stage there are two sections.

→ CENTRAL IDEA
→ BRANCHES + BOI

→ CENTRAL IDEA

If the chat or conference is well made, the speaker will begin by explaining his or her purpose and what he or she hopes to achieve.

It should also provide an initial general overview of everything in the session. If the speaker makes this introduction, we can start to work on our central image, which will surely be closely related to any of his words. On the other hand, if the speaker gives an overview about the subject that he or she will discuss, then he or she is giving us the BOI we need to create the mental diagram.

Part of the challenge in this phase is that the speaker may not make this brief introduction. So we have to pay a lot of attention in the beginning to know exactly if he or she is giving this overview, or if he or she is going directly into the presentation.

→ BRANCHES + BOI

Perhaps this section should be called search and capture ideas, since it is very similar to a hunt. While listening to the speaker, we have to separate the wheat from the chaff, search for useful ideas to build branches, and understand the relationship between them. At the same time, you should realize that the ideas exposed by the lecturer are forming the BOI naturally. Taking notes is a matter of attention and interest. If you think of it as a mental diagram you will be saving time and effort, and you will avoid the frustration that comes when you leave class without understanding anything.

The only challenge in note taking is capturing the presentation's internal structure.

Useful Tips

GOOD EXAMPLES

The speaker may add plenty of examples to illustrate the concepts discussed. These examples are important because they are usually specific explanations and they are highly mnemonic. His examples may make you think of others that are more closely related or more known, and these are equally or more important than the speaker's, so you should assign them their own branches in your mental diagram.

I REMEMBER WHEN . . .

A phenomenon that happens sometimes is that the speaker is going out on a limb and explains things that are of no interest to us. We must know how to distinguish what is useful: at the end of the day, keep in mind that a speaker is often required to fill a set time for the talk.

"FLASHBACK"

I have also frequently observed that the speech is not linear like a book, but there is a constant "flashback" like in some films. This happens because the speaker wants to make constant connections to what he stated before or at other times during the lecture because he forgot to mention an important related issue. You have to pay attention to these sudden changes. Otherwise you will lose some of your work. Follow him and jump with him from branch to branch; do not let him get away!

👁 Exercise number 2: **Wildlife in the savanna**

To train for classes and lectures, there is a way to practice and have fun at the same time by using documentaries. There has to be a documentary type that you particularly tend to enjoy. I like those that deal with space and history. This practice consists of taking notes by making a mental diagram of a documentary on a subject that you like. Choose the documentary, imagine you are at a conference, and create its mental diagram at the same time. Doesn't that sound fun?

HOW CAN MENTAL DIAGRAMS HELP ME WITH NOTE-TAKING?

- Develop the mental abilities of classification, categorization, and accuracy.
- Free your attention and mental clarity.
- Gather complex data in an integrated manner.
- Learning objectives are achieved quickly.
- Permanent and easily accessible records are created.

12 The Business

Much of our life is spent working. The working environment can give us great satisfaction and also generate problems. Greater efficiency in the tasks we carry out can be an important element of our well-being at work. In this chapter we will see that by using creativity, mental diagrams can help us overcome challenges.

- **Glue that does not stick**

- **Houston, we have a problem**

- **The creative process**

- **Creative thinking in mental diagrams**

- **Projects, reports, and conferences**

■ Glue that does not stick

In the 3M laboratories there was a researcher who had a serious problem: he had spent much of their budget, and several months of work, making glue that did not stick. Sooner or later he would be accountable to his supervisor, and he did not know what to say. If only the glue had had another problem, like it hardened, smelled, or had impurities, but it just did not meet its main function of sticking. To be more exact, it did glue a bit but not enough to keep two things together; its gluey power was very little. What use could a product with these features have? Desperate, he confided in a coworker who tried to comfort him; he was young and would surely find another job. Suddenly, the young researcher pointed to a note and asked his colleague what it was. The colleague turned and said, "A reminder. I tape paper notes and hang them to remember important things I have to do." This response came as a thunderbolt to our young scientist friend. He got up close to the note and looked hypnotized. Do you know what we are talking about yet? Yes, the famous yellow self-adhesive Post-it® notes.

■ Houston, we have a problem

Even if you are not one of the researchers at 3M, more than once you must have had a problem you wanted to solve but did not know how. Part of the challenge is that there are situations in which there is no single solution, but rather a range of possibilities, and it is very difficult to know which one is correct. Imagine the faces of the Apollo XIII technical crew when over their headphones they heard the famous phrase "Houston, we have a problem." In 3M's case there was a clear solution that had to do with the new glue. The formula could have been changed, or the product could have been rejected, but no one thought something different, and that is one of the keys to creativity, finding innovative ideas to solve complex problems.

You may not agree with me, but I think that creativity is desirable. Thanks to it, we can now enjoy a range of goods that were once unthinkable, such as the phone or the Internet. Someone saw a problem, the inability to remotely communicate quickly and efficiently, and to solve this problem he created a myriad of devices to try to solve it.

And creativity is not only present in products; it is also in scientific advances and in many arts, such as literature, film, or music. Arranging musical notes to express a feeling is a whole display of creativity.

■ The creative process

There have been many studies on creativity that resulted in the discovery of several phases or stages that usually take place during the creative process:

1. IMMERSION

People who develop a creative solution usually spend long periods immersed in the problem. I am sure that our 3M researcher spent countless hours reviewing his glue's formula and trying to find out what went wrong.

2. INCUBATION

Creative solutions often come about when the person is no longer actively working on the problem. During this period, the person recovers from the fatigue brought on by immersion. At this stage the brain is still working, not consciously but unconsciously, even during dreams. If I close my eyes I can see the poor researcher taking long solitary walks in the park with his head down and shuffling his feet.

3. ENLIGHTENMENT

Sometimes, people involved in the creative process say they see something, like a signal, and then they arrive at the solution. It is interesting to note that often the solution arrives by means of a visual sensation. In the case of Post-it® notes, our investigator had a vision upon seeing the taped note, and somehow he made a "creative association" that led to solving the problem.

4. REFINEMENT

Reaching enlightenment is not the end of the process, since much remains to be refined. The idea must be worked on and tested until it finally appears that the solution is correct. The 3M employee would have had to do many tests until he created the Post-it® as we know it, and he would have had to convince several executives that his proposal was good.

■ Creative thinking within mental diagrams

Glimpsing into the general theory of mental diagrams we can see that these are actually a manifestation of the total creative thinking process. Mental diagrams are totally suited to the creative process because they require all the skills commonly associated with creativity:

- Imagination, association, and flexible ideas

In the Post-it example we can see that all three elements are present. At some point the protagonist was flexible enough to think that glue could serve a different purpose. He was also flexible enough to create an unusual association: glue - note - tape. And finally, he imagined a new product: self-adhesive notes.

■ Projects, reports, and conferences

If you entered the working world a while back, you may have noticed that the business world is not an exact science and there are no unique solutions. You had to constantly use your full potential to solve all types of problems. Based on your ability to respond, you will either be well valued at the company or you will be invited to go use your limited capabilities elsewhere. Undoubtedly, it would be beneficial to add a good dose of creativity to your work performance. And as you saw, mental diagrams can provide you the flexibility, imagination, and association to find creative solutions.

In this chapter dedicated to business, we will look at three applications that involve the creative process:

→   CREATING PROJECTS
→   MAKING REPORTS
→   CONFERENCES

→   CREATING PROJECTS

The business world is based on buying and selling products. Sometimes we are buyers and other times sellers. Often the product is already done and the solution has a name. However, other times we have to create a solution tailored to the client, and this is where a project has to be developed. The client can be either external or internal. For an external client, a high degree of adaptation is needed to present the project in a clear and coherent manner, so that the client senses that every consideration has been taken into account. If it is an internal client, we follow the same path to present a solution tailored to his needs. In both situations we will have to organize a lot of information and we have to find creative solutions using the elements we have available. As you can see, developing a project by creating mental diagrams shares many things in common with the creative process that we described earlier in this chapter, so this concept will not be difficult to grasp.

Stages of project development through mental diagrams
The application of mental diagrams in creating a project has the added bonus of generating several creative ideas that can lead to new solutions. Here are the steps to follow:

1. CENTRAL IMAGE

Like all mental diagrams, we first visualize a figure that represents the project as a whole. Remember that the more details you include in the central image, the easier the associations will appear.

2. BRAINSTORM

Once we have the central image in the center of a large sheet (preferably size A3) we brainstorm. For a maximum of twenty minutes you must let the ideas flow freely as quickly as possible. At this stage, working quickly stimulates creativity and makes you include ideas that may seem absurd but are important in the creative process. Respect such ideas because they are often essential to breaking those limitations imposed on us by the left hemisphere.

3. FIRST RECONSTRUCTION

Take a break and allow your brain to rest because the branching associations that you made in the previous phase could easily reach one hundred. After the break, start organizing and prioritizing ideas according to the basic ordering ideas (BOI). Sort, link, and discover associations, even if they seem absurd. As we saw, the more unconventional the idea, the more interesting it can turn out to be.

4. INCUBATION OF IDEAS

As noted above, creative ideas often appear unexpectedly when the brain is relaxed, perhaps when you are out for a walk, sleeping, or dreaming. Throughout history, great thinkers have used these processes to find their creativity. Famous muses are no other than the unexpected creative spark encountered in moments that are completely unrelated to creative activity.

5. SECOND RECONSTRUCTION

After the incubation process, the brain has a new take on the first mental diagram, so it will help to make a second diagram based on the first. During this reconstruction, you can add ideas and thoughts that accumulated during incubation. In this stage you need to consider all the information collected and integrated into the different diagrams so that you are able to create an ample mental diagram.

6. FINAL STAGE

This is the stage that corresponds to the launch. Surely there will be changes along the way, unexpected twists or unforeseen limitations, but by creating a mental diagram you will be able to have breakthroughs.

Natural fragrances

I have participated in many projects, but one that was particularly interesting was about natural fragrances. There is an increasingly growing tendency to consume natural products. As a result, a company evaluated creating a line of natural soaps. This company was already involved in the chemical sector, but not specifically in cosmetics. Before getting into this market, the company decided to draft a detailed project on the topic. Mental diagrams were used since there was little time and a quick response was needed.

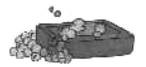

As in all projects, a central image was sought. This image was quite complex and it clearly projected the idea that they had of the product and the type of consumer. A sketch was made followed by a brainstorming session. At first, there were about seventy branches. As you can imagine, we had to cover an entire wall with paper for this project. The diagram below is a partial reproduction of some branches:

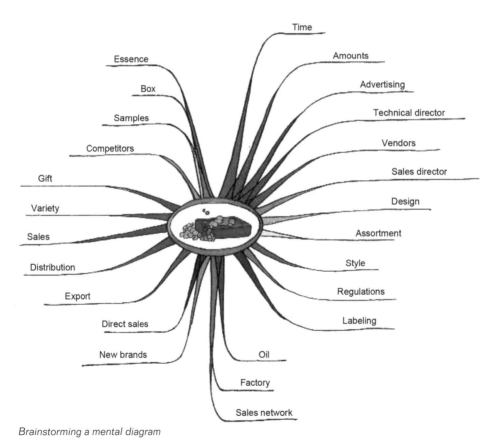

Brainstorming a mental diagram

After a lunch break, we went back to sorting. We moved some of the branches and created the BOI. The result was this:

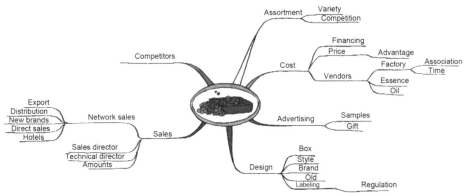

Mental diagram with BOI

If you look closely at this mental diagram, you will notice one thing: there are basic ordering ideas that are almost empty. This was an indication that there were whole areas we did not know or did not have in mind (competitors, marketing, and assortment). We discussed the importance of these areas and realized that they were essential to developing this project. The idea was good, but we were completely unfamiliar with the market, and this was evidenced by the lack of information about the competitors. On the other hand, the assortment had not been given a lot of thorough consideration because no one had previous experience in marketing these products. Advertising was another unknown area, because the company did not directly advertise its industrial chemicals. This diagram had to be expanded by developing the most deficient branches.

As you can imagine, the project was lengthy. After the incubation period, new branches and new questions appeared. An interesting creative element that came up was the idea that the technical director and the sales director should work together. In meetings, they had very different

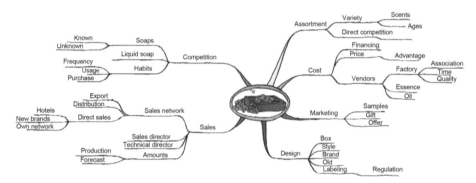

Expanded mental diagram.

points of view about the product; it seemed as though they each saw it with different eyes. Thanks to the mental diagram they were able to understand the project as a whole and decided to cooperate so that the project would grow in a balanced way.

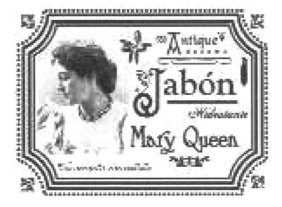

Label sample that was prepared for the project ("Antique Jabon" indicates "antique soap.")

◉ Exercise number 1: The website

I recently participated in a project to develop a website. During the first meeting I noticed that there were some ideas, but nothing had been decided. I suggested working with mental diagrams and the results were excellent. Now imagine that you had to make your own web page. As you can see, it is a complicated project, but doesn't it sound interesting? Go for it!

WHAT CAN MENTAL DIAGRAMS PROVIDE FOR PROJECT DEVELOPMENT?

- Apply every creative thinking skill.
- Generate great mental energy as you delve into the problem.
- Visualize multiple items at once, thus increasing creative and integrative association.
- Increase the possibility of achieving new insights.

→ MAKING REPORTS

In business, making reports is essential. Reports usually encompass elements that you have researched, process results, or sales information. Few companies have standardized reports because doing so would create inflexibility and it would impede presentations from adapting to each situation. In my experience, reports take up a lot of work and in the end you are left not knowing what you did right or wrong, or if it was well reviewed. Well, those are excellent reasons to use the least amount of time possible and present reports in a clear and concise way.

Mental diagrams can say a lot about reports. We already know the methodology, so we simply have to consider a few nuances.

Phases for report preparation

1. CENTRAL IMAGE

At this point, it is important to visualize the central figure as the report's objective. Whenever written information is presented there is a hidden wide-ranging goal. In this case you have to be able to see what you aim to show through the report. You may want to demonstrate that the 3 for the price of 2 offer has yielded no results. In this case, visualize an image that summarizes this idea. Associating the objective to the drawing is crucial to developing a coherent report.

2. BRAINSTORMING

Once there is a clear objective, proceed to brainstorm as quickly as possible. Let there be associations among all kinds of events, issues, statistics, dates, names, etc. This is a good time to create drawings based on this information because drafting a report requires many visual elements.

3. ORGANIZATION

Following the structure of a mental diagram, proceed to sort using the BOI. Facts may show up in two places at once. Include both, but put an arrow that indicates the relationship between them. It is not necessary for the diagram to include exact information that will be part of the finalized report (numbers and figures), just references. Organize it well because it will create the different sections of the report.

4. SEQUENCE AND INFORMATION

Now you must determine what order you will give the branches. Think of how you would write the information in a linear order, so it is important to enumerate the order in which the branches will appear in the report. Once you make this list, find the information on the branches that you will need in detail. For instance, on a branch there could be "annual sales" or "product." So find the annual sales and keep them on hand, or find a technical description of the product to include it when the time comes.

5. WRITE UP

The last thing left to do is write. You should start the report with the central image that clearly explains the purpose of the report. Then all you have to do is write the contents branch by branch, taking into account all the information you gathered. Lastly, go back to the central image and write the objective's result, clearly bringing together its most important points.

Exercise number 2: The unexpected report

Have you been wanting to propose changes, improvements, or a project to your boss for some time? He may have sent you away saying something like "hmm . . . interesting, make a report and I will get back to you." From experience I know that this report never gets made, but here is your chance to actually do it. Follow the steps of making a mental diagram and show your boss your results, then see his face!

HOW CAN MENTAL DIAGRAMS HELP CREATE REPORTS?

- Eliminate the stress and suffering caused by disorganization, fear of failure, and "writer's block."
- Considerably reduce the time required to prepare, organize, and draft a report.
- Allow data processing to be done analytically as well as creatively.
- Get a direct, organized, and structured report.

→ CONFERENCES

Recently I was having coffee with a friend who is a psychotherapist. Talking to her I thought it might be a good idea to have her participate in one of my lectures. She looked puzzled and said it sounded interesting but she would have to think it over. We met the following week and she explained that she very much appreciated the offer but she would not be participating. Then she mentioned that it was not because she was afraid to speak in public, which indicated to me that she was in fact afraid to speak in public. This fear is much more common than we tend to think, even among professionals (like my friend) who make a living talking to people. Can mental diagrams help in public speaking? Yes they can, and in fact that is one of their applications that I use most often. Using mental diagrams you can prepare a clear, effective, and interesting lecture. The flexibility of mental diagrams is a great advantage to lecturers. If during the lecture, a question that you had set aside for later comes up, you can easily jump to that branch and answer it without a problem. Once the issue is resolved you can go back to the branch where you left off or move on to the next. Also, if you feel that you are running out of time, or you have extra time, you can adjust your lecture by eliminating or expanding branches accordingly.

Steps to creating a mental diagram for a conference

1. Continuing with the mental diagrams principles we have to look for the central image to represent our conference.
2. The following step is brainstorming: find all the associations that come to mind and are related to the topic.
3. Look at the mental diagram again and start reorganizing the information through the main branches and less important branches.

Here you can add any new words and associations that come to mind. Once it is clear, estimate the duration of speaking material you have. One way of doing this is by assigning one minute to each word, so if you have fifty words in a mental diagram you have roughly a fifty-minute lecture.

4. Look at the diagram again and trim it a little. Get rid of any items that are not really useful or that add nothing interesting to the topic. At this point you should assign color codes to the BOI; a single glance should tell you the issues that you prepared. Also put signs indicating jokes or anecdotes, transparencies for the projector, questions to ask, or examples. Make it appealing, tasteful, and include items that may be interesting.

5. Now, just as with drafting reports, assign an order to the branches and list them to remind yourself of their priority in the presentation.

6. Finally, assign the amount of time you want to use to expand each branch and write it down, and you will see how simple it is to make a successful presentation.

Exercise number 3: **Soulful**

You may have had to try to persuade attendees at a meeting or conference. As you may have noticed, you cannot get very far by simply improvising. Next time, try making a mental diagram for a conference. Follow the steps explained above and remember that both of your hemispheres have to be working at the same time; your words also have to be visual and contain emotion. Try it—the results are guaranteed.

HOW CAN MENTAL DIAGRAMS HELP IN PREPARING FOR A CONFERENCE?

- Facilitate and increase eye contact with the audience.
- Allow the speaker to meet the needs of his or her audience and make an accurate time estimate.
- Utilize a wide range of mnemonic devices.
- Allow greater freedom of movement.

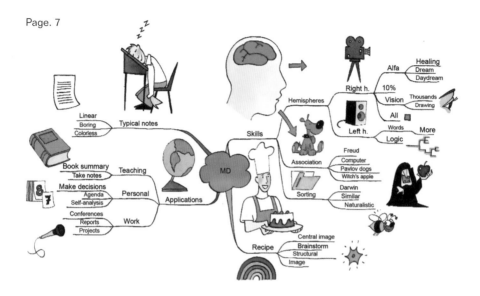

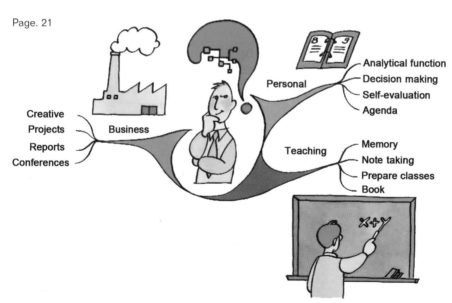

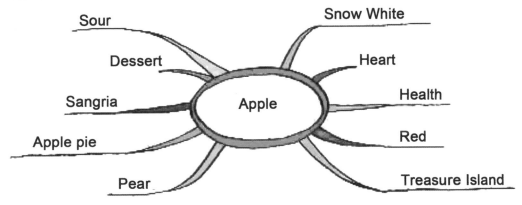

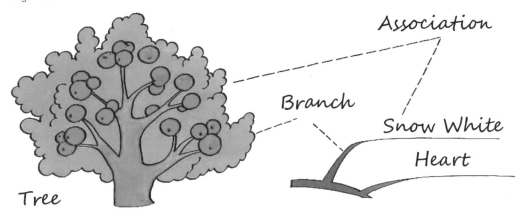

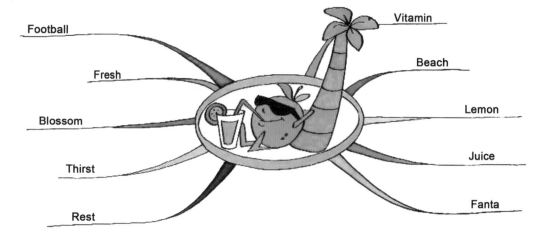

Football
Fresh
Blossom
Thirst
Rest
Vitamin
Beach
Lemon
Juice
Fanta

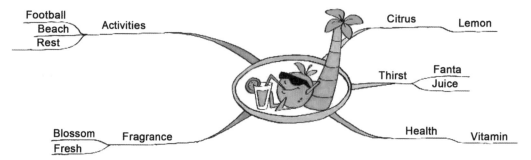

Football
Beach
Rest
Activities

Citrus
Lemon

Thirst
Fanta
Juice

Blossom
Fresh
Fragrance

Health
Vitamin

Page. 114

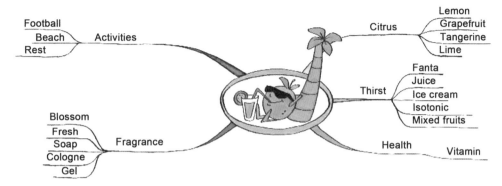

Page. 139

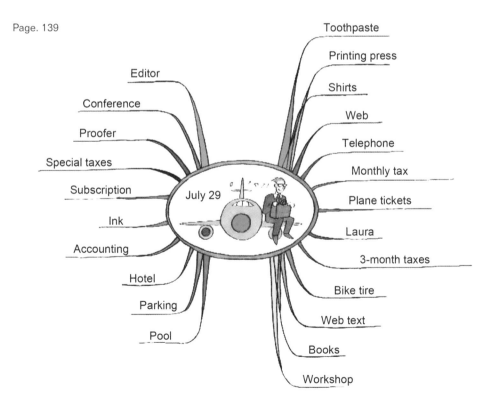

Page. 140

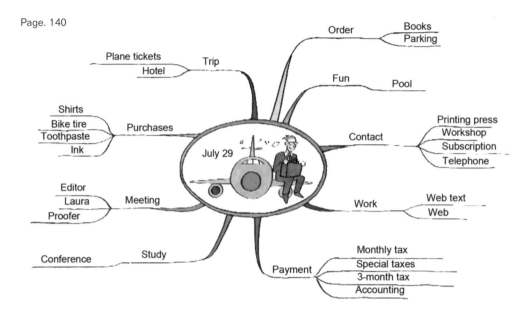

Page. 145

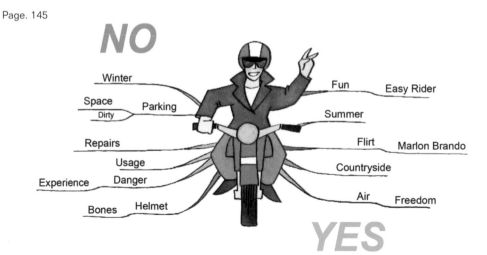

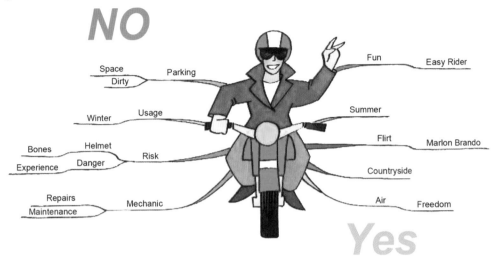

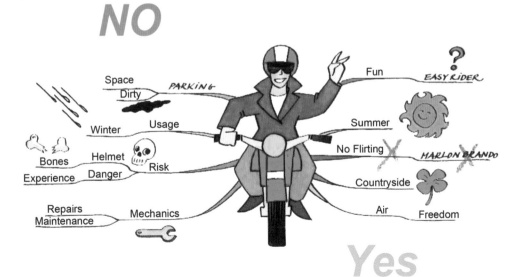

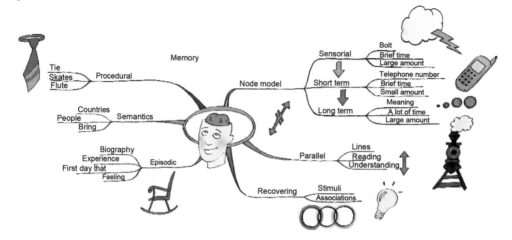

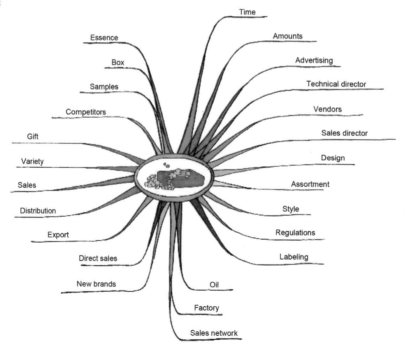

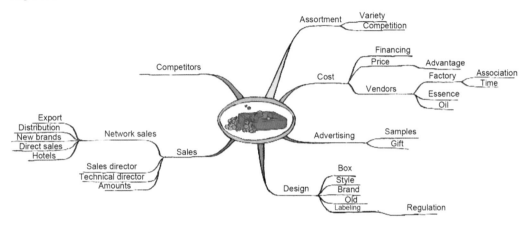

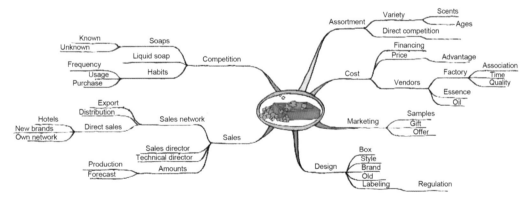